HYPNOSIS
FOR VAGINISMUS TREATM
The Importance of Psoas M

MURAT ULUSOY, MD. Clin. Ps

CİNİUS YAYINLARI

Moda Caddesi Borucu Han No: 20 Daire: 504-505
Kadıköy 34710 İstanbul
Tel: (216) 5505078
http://www.ciniusyayinlari.com
iletisim@ciniusyayinlari.com

MURAT ULUSOY, MD. Clin. Psyc. MA.

HYPNOSIS
FOR VAGINISMUS TREATMENT
THE IMPORTANCE OF PSOAS MUSCLES

FIRST PRINT: January, 2021

Address:
Türkmen Mah. Atatürk Bulv. No. 68/3 Kat 3
D. 6 Kuşadası – Aydın - Turkey
Cell & Whatsapp: +90 505 911 21 51
Web: www.drulusoy.com
Telegram: https://t.me/vajinismus
E-mail: dr_ulusoy@hotmail.com

HYPNOSIS

FOR VAGINISMUS TREATMENT

THE IMPORTANCE OF PSOAS MUSCLES

The path to solution in three phases and one and a half days

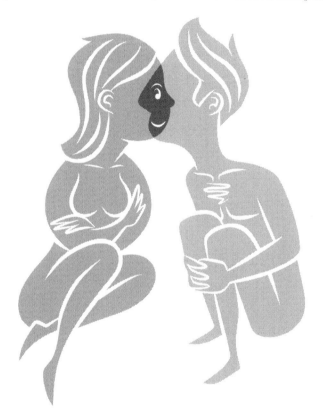

*"The mind does what it imagines and believes.
The rest are details for the mind..."*

MURAT ULUSOY, MD. Clin. Psyc. MA

⊃ Cinius Yayınları

To my high school sweetheart and wife Funda,
To my beloved son Kutay,
To Mom and Dad...

WHO IS DR. MURAT ULUSOY?

I was born in 1969 in Nazilli, where I also completed my education from primary school through high school. In 1986 I scored enough points to attend the Faculty of Pharmacy at Aegean University but I did not get enrolled because of the love I had for medicine. And I was able to get into Thrace University Medical Faculty in 1987, from where I graduated in 1993.

I came across hypnosis during my years at the faculty and since then, I have been working on it within the context of therapy. Together with the Medical Hypnosis Association, I conducted trainings at Yeditepe University, Istanbul Aydın University and Üsküdar University. I am currently the manager of Üsküdar University Traditional and Complementary Medicine Application and Research Center, and I also provide training on Medical Hypnosis at the same university. I have made many presentations at international hypnosis congresses, and I also actively participated in the establishment of hypnosis associations all around Turkey.

In 2007, I completed the training on therapy provided by the Psychotherapy Institute.

I am currently working on vaginismus treatment with The Dr. **Ulusoy Method** (Presented at the 12th European Hypnosis Congress – ESH 2011 Congress). **The Dr. Ulusoy Method is a treatment method that is able to reach a solution in three phases and in one and a half days on average** (Also known as the Three Phase Method).

There is also the Hypnosis Induction Technique, which I call The Dr. **Ulusoy Hypnosis Induction Technique**, which **takes the subject under hypnosis in one to three minutes and which tests the auditory – visual – tactile structures**, and which I had presented at various congresses.

The areas on which I provide trainings are,
1. Hypnosis Induction technique
2. Hypnotic Phenomena
3. Mutual Hypnosis
4. Weight and Hypnosis
5. Hypnotherapy in sexual problems – Vaginismus, Premature Ejaculation, Erectile Dysfunction, Orgasm problems
6. Hypnotic Age Regression
7. Ericksonian Hypnosis
8. Hypnotherapy for Depression Treatment
9. Hypnotherapy for Panic Attack
10. Hypnotherapy for Anxiety
11. Hypnotherapy for Phobias
12. Hypnotherapy for Education
13. Hypnotherapy for Gynecological Diseases and Childbirth

My primary area of concern is vaginismus treatment. In the treatment of vaginismus, I use my own method and allocate special time for each patient and provide one-on-one therapy.

I have focused my studies on a new treatment approach/theory. Below is a brief description.

DR. ULUSOY THERAPY THEORY

1. It targets the human mind and the working mechanisms of the conscious and the subconscious.
2. It contains healthy nutrition and exercising for the body and mind to be healthy, to be prepared for therapy (For treatments other than vaginismus).
3. It is problem and emotions oriented.
4. After identifying the problem, it formulizes the problem via the foursome model (Cognitive – Behaviorist – Dynamic – Existentialist).
5. As the therapy for the problem, it utilizes the "Suggestion, Archetype and Symbol" approach that mainly targets the subconscious, "Smart Intelligence."
6. Its aim is to quickly change the emotions, thoughts and behaviors that disturb the patient both psychologically and psychosomatically.

With this theory, my greatest wish is to provide a more humane therapy approach toward mankind, who is actually perfect in his essence.

TRAİNİNGS, CONGRESS PRESENTATİONS AND CERTİFİCATES

1. Thrace University Medicine Faculty Diploma
2. Yeditepe University Hypnosis-1 Course Training Certificate
3. Yeditepe University Hypnosis-2 Course Training Certificate
4. Yeditepe University Hypnosis-3 Course Training Certificate
5. Providing trainings on "Hypnosis and Induction techniques," "Ericksonian Hypnosis," "Catathymia and Hypnosis," and "Hypnotherapy for Vaginismus Treatment" at the medical hypnosis courses at Yeditepe University.
6. Certificate of Appreciation for the trainings I provide at Yeditepe University.
7. Certificate of Attendance for the 1st Medical Hypnosis Congress of Yeditepe University.
8. Certificate of Appreciation from Yeditepe University and The Medical Hypnosis Association for my contributions at the 1st Medical Hypnosis Congress.
9. Poster presentation on Hypnotherapy for Vaginismus Treatment during the 1st Medical Hypnosis Congress.
10. Certificate of Attendance for Dr. Tahir Özakkaş's "Hypnosis Treatment in Anxiety Disorders" workshop.
11. Certificate of Attendance for Dr. Cenk Kiper's "Hypnosis Treatment in Sexual Problems" workshop.
12. Certificate of Attendance for Prof. John G. Watkins' "Ego State Therapy" workshop.
13. Certificate of Attendance for Prof. Peter Bloom's "Ericksonian Hypnotherapy" workshop.
14. Certificate of Attendance for Prof. Peter Bloom's "Trance Induction Techniques in Hypnosis" workshop.
15. Certificate of Attendance for Austrian psychotherapist and hypnotherapist Prof. Matthias Mende's "Hypnotherapy in Emotional Needs" workshop.

16. Certificate of Attendance for the "Nonverbal Hypnosis" workshop of Prof. Shaul Livnay, President of European Hypnosis Union.

17. Certificate of Attendance for the workshop of Dr. Albert Schmierer, President of German Dental Hypnosis Association.

18. Certificate of Attendance for Asst. Prof. Psychiatrist Ali Babaoğlu's "Catathymic Imaginative Life" workshop.

19. Attendance as lecturer at Haymana 2004 Applied Medical Hypnosis and Hypnotherapy Training.

20. Attendance as lecturer at Haymana 2005 Advanced Medical Hypnosis and Hypnotherapy Training.

21. Given seminar on Medical Hypnosis and its position in Turkey for the Department of Psychiatry of Adnan Menderes University Medical Faculty.

22. Took part in the organization committee of the 2nd Medical Hypnosis Congress in 2005, where I have been honored with a certificate and a plaque.

23. Participated in the "The Creative Process in Psychotherapy and Hypnotherapy" workshop of Prof. Peter Bloom at the 2ns Medical Hypnosis Congress.

24. Conducted two workshops on "Hypnosis Induction Techniques and Deepening the Trance" for the congress attenders at the 2nd Medical Hypnosis Congress, giving poster and verbal presentations on hypnotherapy in vaginismus treatment.

25. During the 2nd Medical Hypnosis Congress with local and foreign attendance, I have made the declaration that the "Seesaw Effect" is the secondary erection problem that can be seen in the man during vaginismus treatment, and that visualization should be used as the final step of the treatment and that this has been given the name "Simulation Method."

26. Attendance at Gyn. Surgeon Bülent Uran's "5-PATH, Analytic Hypnotherapy, and Hypnosis in Gynecology" workshop.

27. Provided trainings in sixteen workshops at Medical Hypnosis Courses-1, 2 and 3 at Yeditepe University on topics such as *Ericksonian Hypnosis, Hypnosis Induction techniques, Cathatymia-Hypnosis, Hypnosis and Hypnotherapy for Vaginismus Treatment* and I still continue to do so.

28. Provided a training on "Hypnosis Induction techniques" at the Clinical and Applied Hypnosis Association (2005).

29. Provided training on "Clinical Hypnosis" for the Ankara Hypnosis Group (2002).

30. Provided training on "Vaginismus and Hypnotherapy" for the Ankara Hypnosis Group (2003).

31. Certificate and plaque for the 200-hour Holistic Psychotherapy Theoretical Training by Dr. Tahir Özakkaş at the Psychotherapy Institute.

32. Certificate of Attendance for the 8th Psychoanalysis Congress and for the 3-day "Therapeutic Factors in Psychotherapy and Patient Approaches" workshop of Psychiatrist Vamık Volkan during the same congress.

33. Application, Competency and Trainer certificates from Yeditepe University Dentistry Faculty, Basic Medical Sciences Department and Medical Hypnosis Association.

34. Certificate of Attendance for Prof. Peter Krijger's "Hypnosis combined with body-work for the treatment of posttraumatic stress" workshop at the 3rd National Medical Hypnosis Congress.
35. Certificate of Attendance for Prof. Lucia Baricevic-Rademaker's "How to combine modern and neo-classic hypnotherapy for fast results" workshop at the 3rd National Medical Hypnosis Congress.
36. Certificate of Attendance for Specialist Psychologist Tuncay Özer's "Hypnosis Applications in Psychology" workshop at the 3rd National Medical Hypnosis Congress.
37. Certificate of Attendance for Asst. Prof. Osman Özcan's "Practical Hypnosis Applications" workshop at the 3rd National Medical Hypnosis Congress.
38. Certificate of Attendance for Dr. Ali Özden Öztürk's "Conscious Hypnosis Applications" workshop at the 3rd National Medical Hypnosis Congress.
39. Certificate of Attendance for Prof. Shaul Livnay's "An integrative to stage model of hypnotherapy with anxiety disorders" workshop at the 3rd National Medical Hypnosis Congress.
40. Certificate of Attendance for Prof. Matthias Mende's "Hypnotic communication with the symptom in psychosomatic patients: establishing contact, negotiation, integration" workshop at the 3rd National Medical Hypnosis Congress.
41. Provided visual presentation on *Hypnotic Phenomena*, poster presentation on *Mayalama Method for Vaginismus Treatment*, and workshop on *hypnotic induction techniques*. Also acted as session moderator and panelist during lectures. Awarded with a plaque for contributions during the 3rd National Medical Hypnosis Congress.
42. Received 600-hour Holistic Psychotherapy and Clinical Hypnosis Training containing behavioral, cognitive, dynamic and existential models from psychiatrist, psychotherapist and hypnotherapist Dr. Tahir Özakkaş.
43. Received training from Prof. Walter Bongratz on Psychosomatic Diseases and Hypnosis.
44. Conveyed personal "Hypnosis Applications" during the Psychology Days at Muğla University.
45. Participated in the 5th Medical Hypnosis Congress in 2008 with verbal presentation "Dr. Ulusoy Method in Vaginismus Treatment" at Istanbul Aydın University.
46. Provided presentation on "Main Factors Influencing Vaginismus Treatment; twenty main causes and four new definitions" at the 6th International Medical Hypnosis Congress in 2009.
47. Provided presentation on "Dr. Ulusoy Hypnosis Induction Technique" and "Dr. Ulusoy Vaginismus Treatment Method" and shared retrospective analysis and survey results for 450 cases at the 12th ESH (European Hypnosis Congress) in 2011; thus reducing the treatment duration to twenty-four hours.
48. Provided verbal presentation on "Weight and Hypnosis," "Vaginismus Treatment" and "Dr. Ulusoy Hypnosis Induction Technique" at the 8th International Medical Hypnosis Congress in 2012 at Üsküdar University.
49. Presented the "Dr. Ulusoy Hypnosis Induction Technique" to the members of Ankara Hypnosis Association.

50. Participated in Assen Allaaddin's Hypnotherapy Training at the Psychotherapy Institute in 2013.
51. Participated in the Sexual Therapy Training of CITEB (Sexual Therapy Institute of Educational Sciences) in 2013.
52. Attended Prof. G. D. Benedittis' "Hypnotic Mind" workshop at the Psychotherapy Institute in 2014.
53. Attendance Certificate for the 450-hour "Family Consulting Training" approved by Süleyman Demirel University.
54. Translated "The Oxford Handbook of Hypnosis: Theory, Research, and Practice" that is the basic handbook of hypnosis that also includes latest literature reviews. It was published in 2015 by the Psychotherapy Institute.
55. Published Turkish version of the book "Hypnosis for Vaginismus Treatment" in 2015.
56. Provided a verbal presentation and workshop for "Three phases and one and a half days in Vaginismus Treatment – Dr. Ulusoy Method" and the "5 – BK Model" at the International Anatolian Twin Congress On Neuroscience and Sexual Health in Istanbul in 2015.
57. Attended Prof. G. D. Benedittis' "Miracle Healings; Wake up your Inner Healer" workshop at the Psychotherapy Institute in 2016.
58. Received "Hypnosis Application Equivalence Certificate" from the Ministry of Health in 2016.
59. Conducted "Hypnomeditation; Wake up your Inner Healer" workshop at the 2nd Eurasia Positive Psychology Congress.
60. Received "Hypnosis Unit" license from the Ministry of Health.
61. Completed postgraduate study on Clinical Psychology at Esentepe University in 2018. Presented "Hypnosis Application for Vaginismus Treatment" as graduation project.
62. TedX Gölbaşı Talk on Social Responsibility in Vaginismus, 2018.
63. Attended Gaby Golan's workshop in 2018.
64. Attended Catherine Potter's workshop in 2018.
65. Attended Mehdi Fathi's workshop in 2018.
66. Provided presentation on "Enhanced Sexual Satisfaction" at Üsküdar University 1st Clinical Hypnosis Days Symposium.
67. Provided presentation on "Hypnosis in Vaginismus and Psoas Muscles" at 11th Congress of Turkish Hypnosis Association in 2018.
68. Founded CITEHIPAK (Sexual Therapy and Hypnosis Academy).
69. Provided presentation on "Enhanced Sexual Satisfaction" during the Novelties in Sexual Therapy Event at Üsküdar University.
70. TedX Üsküdar University Talk on Enhanced Sexual Satisfaction.
71. Provided presentation on "Hypnosis for Vaginismus and the Psoas Muscle" at the 1st Asia Hypnosis Congress in Iran in 2019.
72. Provided presentation on "Hypnosis for Vaginismus and the Psoas Muscle" at the 2nd Anatolia Sexual Health and Neuroscience Congress in 2019.

Offered free of charge support during 2005 – 2006 for vaginismus patients via the Yahoo! group. Provided treatment for 146 vaginismus patients as a social responsibility project.

Applied "Weight and Hypnosis" project on himself during 2012 – 2013 March and succeeded in coming down from 317lbs to 165lbs…

CONTENTS

CHAPTER 1

VAGINISMUS IN ALL ASPECTS

CHAPTER 2

"DR. ULUSOY METHOD" IN VAGINISMUS TREATMENT

CHAPTER 3

HYPNOSIS AND ITS USE IN VAGINISMUS

CHAPTER 4

CLASSICAL TREATMENT IN VAGINISMUS AND VAGINISMUS DIARIES

CHAPTER 5

USEFUL INFORMATION

CHAPTER 6

REFERENCES AND PHOTOGRAPHS

FOREWORD

Dear Reader,

This book is prepared for the treatment of vaginismus that is frequently seen in Turkey, and it is based on my clinical hypnosis studies and experiences on vaginismus treatment over many years. Many of the definitions and methods you will read here have been created as a compilation of the results of my studies, rather than existing definitions and methods.

I have been dealing with hypnosis since 1991. And since 2004, I have been working exclusively on vaginismus treatments. I have taken part in the founding of many hypnosis associations and I have also contributed to the creation of the Medical Hypnosis Platform. I have been working with the Medical Hypnosis Association and the Conscious Hypnosis Group since 2001, and I also completed my psychotherapy training at the Psychotherapy Institute. I am conducting Medical Hypnosis trainings at Yeditepe University, Istanbul Aydın University and recently at Üsküdar University. I am also the manager of GETIPMER (Traditional and Complementary Medical Center) of Üsküdar University since 2017. I have also offered my translation of the four-volume and academically important book *Hypnosis; Theory, Research, Clinic and Application* which was released by the Psychotherapy Institute Publications for the use of hypnotherapists.

I owe a debt of gratitude for the friends of hypnosis who have helped me arrive to the place I am today. I also sincerely thank the employees of Cinius Publications and especially Ms. Bijen Akgöl, who has provided personal support, and finally to Bora Koçar for the fastidious translation.

I have received strong demand over the years from both my vaginismus patients and also from my fellow therapists for this book to be written. I could have written the book during my first years in vaginismus treatment but if I had done it then, it would not contain my experiences. I know for a fact that the most important things for both the therapist and the patient are experiences and practical information. Today, at the point I have reached in vaginismus treatment, I am happy to be sharing my experiences with you.

In this book, as a first in the World, you will find information declaring that in **vaginismus etiology, it is not the pelvic floor muscles and Kegel Exercises that matter, but that the muscle group creating the real problem is the Psoas Muscles.** *When working with the correct muscle group, the solution can be obtained in a total of three hours of work and between twelve to twenty-four hours with the eclectic and integrative approach.*

In the first publication of the book in 2015, the duration of the treatment had been expressed as one and a half days. In terms of remaining loyal to that edition and to show the development in the treatment method, the same expression has been used throughout the book.

Just as the little bee takes pollens from every flower to produce its unique honey, I am hoping that you will feel the same taste and pleasure while reading this book. Therefore, in effort to ease learning and understanding, the subjects have been written simply, using story-type narration. I can say that this type of transfer has targeted subconscious learning.

This book, which had been published in 2015 in Turkish, has been reviewed during the past five years for the English version, and the subjects on the Psoas Muscles and the Sexual Mind have been added.

I dedicate my book to my mom, dad, my wife Funda, my son Kutay and to all my tutors who have raised me; I could not have been at this position if not for them.

AUGUST 20, 2020 –
DR. ULUSOY, KUŞADASI, TURKEY, 12:30

Web: www.drulusoy.com
Facebook: www.facebook.com/groups/drulusoy
Instagram: dr.ulusoy_klinikhipnoz
E-mail: drmuratulusoy@gmail.com
Cell & Whatsapp: +90 505 911 21 51

WHO CAN BENEFIT FROM THIS BOOK?

The book has been written with multifaceted approach, with many years of experience. It has been structured in eight stages:

1. Vaginismus - Definitions
2. The "Dr. Ulusoy Method" in vaginismus treatment and his contributions
3. Structuring of hypnotherapy-supported vaginismus treatment "5-BK Model – Dr. Ulusoy, 2014" for psychologists and psychiatrists
4. Therapy experiences and stories of patients cured with The Dr. Ulusoy Method
5. Hypnosis Induction, Deepening, and the usage of Clinical Hypnosis in vaginismus
6. Classical approach in vaginismus treatment
7. Vaginismus treatment diaries
8. Exercise experiences and stories on Yahoo! Group by patients seeking classical vaginismus treatment

The first stage is written for both patients and therapists. Stages two through five are prepared for therapists, while two and four are also for informing vaginismus patients about The Dr. Ulusoy Method. Stages six through eight are about the treatments from the patients' viewpoint -mainly those who seek classical treatment or try to find solutions at home- so they also contain teachings and feedback for therapists, and in addition, they also provide comparison of The Dr. Ulusoy Method with classical treatment.

The main reason why patients' stories are included is that they are highly educating. Patient names and locations are withheld, thus concealing their personal information, and their stories have been narrated with their consent. Without your conscious mind even being aware of it, your subconscious will learn about many things with the stories and applications.

TRUE LOVE STORIES - 1

Let's start our book with real life stories…

First Story

A young newlywed couple who got married less than a year ago. They are a perfect match for each other. They had vaginismus problem. We worked together and they went through the intercourse experience. However, the hymen was probably semilunar or circle shaped and there was no bleeding in their experience. In the beginning of the treatment, during the training period, I tell all my patients that four out of ten hymens will not be deformed. Nevertheless, I felt that the man was somewhat bothered with this. I explained to him once again, told him with information from the literature, references and photographs. He said, "Okay," halfheartedly… Less than three months later, I received the information that the man was divorcing his -allegedly- beloved wife because of his hymen-obsessed thoughts.

Second Story

Our 25-year vaginismus patient had tried treatments in the past but when they were all unsuccessful; her twenty-five years had flied by. I asked the man's occupation; "I'm a bicycle repairman," he said, "But I love my wife. Even if we don't have intercourse or a child, I have always remained faithful to her because of the deep love I have for her in my heart, and I never upset her." In the meanwhile, his wife was approving these words in tears.

I gave you two extreme examples. Both couples had married lovingly. One of them had exchanged his love for hymen; the other had protected and grown his love despite everything.

There is a difference of criterion in the two loves. The youth of our time can measure love with factors such as *a momentary liking, physical appearance, social status, materiality, having the same taste in food or music, or having the same habits of travelling and vacations.* When you take these as criteria, problems and disagreements come up in marriages in the following years. Arguments, fights and divorces happen for trivial reasons. Is it love that has ended in such case? If you asked the couples, it is love that has ended. But in reality, we notice that love, which has to be in the foundation of the building, is non-existent and that external factors are perceived and evaluated as love.

True love is the love in the second story. Actually, in its essence is the love that Mevlana feels for Shams[1]. It is *the unification of two souls in a single mind in terms of heart, compassion, and all thoughts and emotions.* And this love is so strong that when Shams left, Mevlana had wept for days, weeks and months. He had felt that a piece inside of him had been torn and gone. He had sought Shams everywhere.

When they say they are in love, this is what I ask the youngsters, "*Does your partner like animals? Does he love humans? Does he help those in hardship, the stranded? Does he love flowers, insects and the creepy crawly? Is he able to convey the love inside him, with compassion and by heart, to his surroundings, to nature, to the people and all creatures? Try to see these. It is not enough just to try to see; test him with events and stories... What reactions does he give at events and stories filled with compassion and heartfelt emotions; take a step back and observe.*

If he can do all this, love that youngster. Love him so much that you never let him go despite everything; like the bicycle repairman. Because he will love you very much and will not let you go no matter what. If such love is in the foundation of the building, the previous things that you had listed as love will be forming the upper floors on this foundation and you will construct a strong building.

If you don't feel the love that Mevlana felt for Shams, walk away. Because that lover will walk away from you at the slightest problem. He will not understand your words, your thoughts or your feelings."

Tell our children and our youth about true heartfelt love with real life stories... As emphasized by mythologist J. Campbell, the things that the young people of our time lack the most are stories. Stories are true, experiences things. When one falls into hardship or struggles, his mind finds solutions via these stories. In a sense, stories are life's guiding maps. They prevent us from making mistakes, or at least, from making the same mistakes over and over again...

---

(1) **TN:** Shams Tabrizi was a Persian poet, who is credited as the spiritual instructor of Mevlana Jalal ad-Dīn and is referenced with great reverence in Mevlana's poetic collection.

"If Mevlana was not able to hold back his sobbing tears for months when he lost Shams, you should also find the lover that will shed tears for you..."

"Come, come again, whoever you are, come anyway,
Heathen or Zoroastrian,
Or idolatrous, come anyway.
Our convent is not one of hopelessness,
Come even if you've broken your penitence a hundred times...
We plant no seed other than love into this earth,
We plant no seed other than love into this spotless field...
Come closer, closer! Come even closer! How long will this wandering last?
If you are I, and I am you, how long will this you versus me last...
Don't look for our grave in the ground after we die!
Our grave is in the hearts of the enlightened."

MEVLANA

CHAPTER 1

VAGINISMUS IN ALL ASPECTS

In this chapter, definitions on vaginismus have been made
from various perspectives, and supported with questions and answers.

VAGINISMUS PATIENTS WANT UNDERSTANDING
RATHER THAN PREJUDICE

THE STORY OF THE WEASEL

A childless married couple was going to the crop field to work, as in any other day.

While they are working, they watch the fight between a snake and a weasel. The mother weasel lets the snake eat her in order to protect her baby, and the snake goes away.

The baby weasel is left there on its own. The woman says, "Poor thing! Let's take it to our house and feed it," and they take it home.

Some time passes by and the couple has a baby. Of course the weasel has grown and has become a part of the family.

One day, the couple needs to rush to the field but the baby is sleeping in the house. "Nothing will happen, we'll be back in an hour," says the man and they take their tools and go to the field. When they come back, they open the door and what do they see! The weasel is walking around the house with its mouth covered in blood.

Upon seeing this, the man goes off the deep end and kills the weasel, hitting it with the shovel in his hand.

Then they look in all the rooms to find the baby. They look to see the baby sound asleep in his room. And when they look around the baby, they see a dead snake and they understand that the weasel had killed the snake to protect the child…

The man falls to his knees and eats himself up, saying," What have I done? How could I do so wrong?"

What did you feel when you read this story?

"Did you feel a pang of sorrow in your heart? Were you sorry? The weasel was wronged just because its name was weasel, right?"

Vaginismus patients are wronged most of the time too... Even their consciouses cannot understand the reactions that they give subconsciously. And most of the time, their husbands don't understand them either. "You don't do it because you don't want to, you don't love me," they say and try to beat them up or even take things all the way to divorce. Since some therapists cannot comprehend the subconscious and emotional structure of the illness, the patients may not be understood by them either. They cannot tell their parents, fearing of being misunderstood or because the topic is a taboo... How could she say that she is unable to do something that her mother can do? Even if she did say, the mother would not understand. The vaginismus patient gradually becomes lonely, withdraws, cries secretly and falls to the bottom day by day...

*Downtrodden weasels! You are **NOT ALONE** anymore! This book was written with a therapy percept and language that understands you, meant to support each of you... Because my experiences have shown that the vaginismus patient starts healing at the moment she feels that she is understood...*

WHAT IS VAGINISMUS?

According to the classical definition, vaginismus is the spasm of the lower 1/3 of vaginal muscles. The penis can never go into the vagina. Finger penetration is not possible. Tampons cannot be placed inside. The ultrasound probe cannot enter. (According to the current psychiatry diagnosis and treatment book, DSM 5 TR, vaginismus is an illness.)

Or, even if the vagina allows finger or tampon penetration, the person has the fear and anxiety of painful intercourse as well as symptoms of panic attack with heart palpitations triggered by medorthophobia and/or first time fright that manifest themselves as contractions and withdrawal at the legs and/or body, backing away in bed, twisting the body left and right, pushing away the spouse, or crying spells.

In addition, in the *vaginismus seen in Turks, the VAGINA IS LOOSE!* Something can go inside easily; there are no contractions at the lower 1/3 of vaginal muscles (Dr. Ulusoy definition – 2005). The actual problem is at the Psoas Muscles.

If you have one or more of the symptoms mentioned above, you are probably unable to have intercourse or you are having difficulty in doing so. In short, we define this as VAGINISMUS or inability to have sexual intercourse. In both options, the person is unable to have gynecological examinations or they struggle a lot. As a paradox, there are also vaginismus patients that are able to have such examinations.

The vaginal muscles having contractions and disallowing penetration, and the contraction/withdrawal of the legs and body can be seen singularly or at the same time.

In primary vaginismus, the first intercourse cannot be experienced. And in secondary vaginismus, sexual intercourse may have been experienced, but after a while, vaginismus may develop with a behaviorist or existentialist mechanism after the woman gets raped or if the husband cheats on her. In our country, it is primary vaginismus that is predominantly observed.

An approach that does not see vaginismus as an illness, sees it as a symptom and cures the symptom. And when you cure the symptom without removing the source of the problem, the penis-vagina relationship may mechanically be realized but you may have problems having pleasure or you may still have contractions and anxieties during this mechanical intercourse. Or, the subconscious may produce different symptoms in the body...

In reality, the woman needs physical, emotional and mental treatment in vaginismus. Therefore, we adopt a holistic approach in our treatments.

VAGINISMUS GENERAL EVALUATION

Despite the fact that we are in the age of information, vaginismus is a nightmare for a considerable number of women. If there is sufficient information, why is vaginismus still seen?

In the past, I had a case where the patient had always had a great dialogue with her father. When she entered puberty, the father had drawn pictures to explain to her the genital structure so that she did not have problems in her first experience. Interestingly, this case came before us as a case of vaginismus.

Apparently, information alone is not sufficient. It is possible to explain this with the working mechanism of the mind. The information experienced, heard or coded with fear in the past, actually resurface during intercourse and the woman thinks that she will feel a lot of pain, have a lot of difficulty. And by believing in this, she creates reactions in a different ego state.

WHAT IS SIMPLE VAGINISMUS?

The data has not been coded as dangerous in the past but the woman lacks sexual experience and knowledge. She is unable to have sexual intercourse due to lack of knowledge. She can easily have intercourse after receiving this information from books or the internet or from her physician. There is no serious fear, state of panic, pushing the spouse away or contractions in simple vaginismus. The existence of such symptoms defines more serious cases of vaginismus.

HOW SHOULD VAGINISMUS BE CLASSIFIED?

In my opinion, classification according to ability of having gynecological examination is wrong. Because while some vaginismus patients are able to have examinations easily, they may still show reactions during intercourse. Therefore, it would be more accurate to make a functional classification with the patient's ability to be observed, touched, penetrated by something, or with the existence of contractions. You may read about my classification based on functionality under the related topic.

VAGINISMUS AND FIRST NIGHT FRIGHT

The first night (Wedding night) fright is a type of fear that fills every girl's mind with imaginary structures ever since childhood. It is a type of fear that is created by hearsay stories suggesting that the first night will be very difficult, that she will feel a lot of pain, she will bleed a lot, that she will be unable to walk or sit after intercourse, that the penis will be stuck inside the vagina, that something like a broomstick will enter her in there, that her pupils will pop out, etc.

This fear is continuously embittered with information received from one's surroundings. And when the first night comes, the mind perceives this imaginate fear as real because it is prone to create its own subjective world. Just as intercourse is about to take place, the mind creates symptoms of panic in the body such as heartthrobs, irregular breathing, contractions, abstinence, pushing away, etc. These symptoms are so elevated that the woman is in a completely different state in that moment. She is experiencing a whole different situation.

If the source of the fear were a real situation, it could be solved with a specific treatment. A hymen problem and the related pain, for example. But as the source of the problem is the mind creating a subjective world for itself after an imaginate process and perceiving this as reality, the problem cannot be solved with a hymen operation or by trying intercourse with anodyne.

The state of self that we call ego symbolizes our daily, momentary state of consciousness. There are lower-selves under our ego, different roles. And under this, there are our subconscious *Shadow Complexes* (Jung) that trigger imaginate fears. These shadow complexes are exactly what we need to work on during vaginismus treatment.

We see that some patients cannot find any solutions even if they apply to different places or different treatments for long durations. The patient does not heal even though the therapist applies or advises her to apply everything that is classically essential in vaginismus treatment.

Here, at this point, we are referring to the fact that the treatment does not reach the necessary points in the mind, and that it cannot remove the existing imaginate fear.

It is also possible for the person to individually overcome this imaginate fear. But this is valid for situations where the fear is at a lower frequency. The person could address the fear with her own will and be successful. But if these fears, these shadow complexes, have been well organized, and if they are at intermediate or higher intensity levels, the person cannot overcome the fear with her own willpower.

And at this point, a good vaginismus treatment is one which not only offers training and vaginal controls, but which essentially removes the fear in the mind, thus providing relaxation. The success rate is quite high in treatments that conform to this trilogy (Dr. Ulusoy congress presentation).

WHAT SHOULD A WOMAN DO WHEN SHE FINDS OUT SHE HAS VAGINISMUS?

The vaginismus woman should start treatment without wasting any time. If she delays for any reason, years will fly by and every intercourse that is tried and unachieved will carry vaginismus to even further depths.

Upon finding out that she has vaginismus; the woman should leave aside her sorrow and explain to her husband that the situation is an illness. At this point, if the man says, "No this is not an illness and you can do it if you want to," or "Let's leave it to time, we'll manage it," it will bring along insolvability. Just as one seeks professional help with other mental and psychological illnesses, vaginismus should also be treated in the same category.

There are cases where the patient solves vaginismus by self-reading or with advice from others who have overcome vaginismus. But it should not be forgotten that these are situations that I have mentioned as simple vaginismus that are actually the *inability to have sexual intercourse due to lack of knowledge*. And they are ten percent of total cases. During the studies we conducted in online groups during 2005 and 2006, we had succeeded in helping 146 women to have sex, out of 1460 group members. All we did was providing information and training. So, we should differentiate between vaginismus and the inability to have sex due to lack of knowledge.

Providing advice such as, "I beat vaginismus, you should do this and that, and you can do it too" in online forums without the supervision of a physician will cause waste of time in real vaginismus cases.

Another problem with such online forums is that hearsay, inaccurate and deficient information is being conveyed in a domino effect because there is no physician control or supervision. And we need to exert extra efforts to correct the wrong information and improper applications with patients who have not been able to solve their problems in online forums before coming to us for treatment.

And another important point is that the man has to refrain from experiences that could cause insecurity or that are forceful.

CAUSES OF VAGINISMUS

What is the cause of your vaginismus?

People face problems because of various reasons. Even though we call the inability to have sexual intercourse as vaginismus in general, it could mostly be caused by fears and anxieties, and continue with involuntary, automatic subconscious gestures such as contraction in your legs or pushing your spouse away in bed, which may be seen singularly or together with the contraction in the vaginal muscles. Your subconscious and your body are affected in four different models.

1. **Behaviorist Model**: There is abuse or a bad sexual experience in the past. Or you may have seen a couple having sexual intercourse while you were a child and you may have perceived the woman's experience as painful and miserable, internalizing the behavior. Another reason is domestic adulterous behavior (Incest).
2. **Cognitive Model**: First night experiences that your friends tell you about like Freddy's nightmares…it will hurt a lot, it will bleed a lot, it will burst, the penis will be stuck inside, etc. Although you have not had a bad experience, these will create negative schemes about sexuality in your subconscious, and these schemes will activate in your future sexual relationships and manifest your involuntary contractions as a subconscious reflex arc. Now your body is not under your control anymore. A faultily programmed autopilot is leading you…
3. **Dynamic Model**: It is a Freudian approach. It could result from problems during the ages of psychological development. It also includes the authoritarian, protective and oppressive structure of the mother, father or other family members. The prohibitions and authority imposed on you by your family and your environment in the past regarding sexuality are important.
4. **Existentialist Model**: You have neither any abuse nor any negative schemes from your upbringing in the past… You may not have any problems in terms of dynamic structure either. But if you still cannot have sexual intercourse, the existentialist model is involved. When we study these couples, we see that the man does not show enough interest in the woman. After one, two or three times, the woman starts an automatic subconscious behavior to express herself to her partner. Her legs tend to cramp up during sex, she

pushes her partner away, runs away from bed, even cries... Without being aware of it, she is making her partner feel her presence.

Your problem could be directly linked to one of these four main causes, or it could be a combination of some or all of them. There, under hypnosis, we get to the bottom of your problem, determine which model or models it fits, and then we provide a suitable approach. Especially if the problem is related to the existentialist model, we teach new approaches where the woman can make her existence felt by her spouse, and we also provide training for the man on showing support and interest to his wife. For instance, if the vaginismus is related to an existentialist model and if we disregard that and try to solve it with behaviorist or cognitive methods, we may succeed and intercourse may take place. But then, the other side of the coin will step in and we will have taken away the woman's self-expression behaviors that she performs by reflex, with subconscious desire. Just as the child feels depressed when his candy is taken away from him, the same mechanism starts working in the woman whom we think we have cured. And in the following time period, the woman experiences worry, depression and anxiety without knowing why. And after that, this will extend to not having pleasure in her relationship, to inability of having orgasms and then to vaginismus resurfacing again...

As opposed to other therapy methods, the inclusion of hypnotherapy to cognitive and behaviorist treatments in vaginismus will increase the success rate due to its ability to provide easier analysis and determination of the model or models, its ability to increase suggestibility, and its ability to provide quick mental intervention to the detected cause...

Moreover,

Although the rate of incidence is reflected as one percent in international literature, in Turkey the rate of vaginismus may go up to ten percent due to the fears and the prohibition of intercourse by the events pushed back into the subconscious. Events pushed back into the subconscious cause the manifestation of leg spasms and fears of feeling aches or pain. In our country, it is a major problem for more women than thought.

OTHER CAUSES OF VAGINISMUS

1. Vaginismus due to contraction of lower vaginal muscles and pelvic floor muscles (1%).
2. Fear and beliefs that ache and pain will be experienced.
3. Having a low pain threshold.
4. A sexual trauma experienced in the past.
5. The psychosomatic effect of an unknown thought or behavior pushed back into the subconscious.
6. Vaginismus developed because of the thought that women are perceived as metas or sexual objects.
7. Staying away from the man in an inappropriate relationship and the vaginismus that develops accordingly.
8. Vaginismus related to the woman's painful or forceful abusive experience on the first night or pre-marriage.
9. Beliefs that sexuality and intercourse are dirty, disgusting or ugly.
10. Exaggerated first-night stories that the woman has heard from her friends.
11. Having used rectal suppositories during childhood.
12. A previous blow or trauma experienced at the genitals.
13. Having been raised with strict sexual prohibitions and taboos.
14. Having unconsciously accumulated sexual knowledge that result in the fear of having too many children to look after could cause vaginismus.
15. False myths such as; the hymen will burst, it will bleed a lot, something like a broomstick will go inside, eyes need to face the ceiling… The hymen does not burst, it deforms. Four out of ten hymens are elastic, they do not bleed, they allow penetration. Even if they do bleed, most hymens would not bleed enough to fill a woman's sanitary pad. It bleeds like a leak and stops.
16. The fear that the penis will be stuck inside and that they will need to go to the hospital in that position, and that they will need an injection to take out the penis. The vagina does not contract in a way that it will lock the penis inside. Let's assume that your vagina squeezes the penis inside (The penis is a spongy structure that fills up with blood). Just as the air changes place when you squeeze a long balloon, the blood in the penis returns to the body and the penis becomes freed from the vagina. In practice, clinically, there cannot be a locking. Locking is only possible in dogs and similar. Because their penis has a 1/3 bone structure at the rear. Their erected penises may be stuck inside.

It is possible to give more examples. When we evaluate these examples, we cannot continue without remembering the saying, "There is really no illness, there is the ill."

What we do is, we first listen to the counselee's story. We evaluate the information they provide at the conscious level. We try to understand what they face during their intercourse trials.

Later, the counselee is informed about hypnosis. Her consent is taken and a pre-session that consists of induction is provided. The aim here is to measure the depth of the trance and to examine her responses to the suggestions.

Between the sessions, the counselee is given homework regarding short-term feedback exercises on the vagina. The problems she faces are discussed in the next session and suggestions regarding those problems are emphasized.

If the vaginismus is due to the contraction of *lower 1/3 of vaginal muscles and the pelvic floor muscles, relaxation techniques and symptom displacement techniques are used to remove muscle contractions.* (In the vaginismus seen in Turks, lower vaginal muscles and pelvic floor muscles are loose.)

If there is fear, or pain, or an underlying event from the past, such events are focused on with hypnoanalysis (Age regression) and the problematic moment is deactivated.

Vaginismus may be seen in any woman at fertile age. It could be experienced in the first try or it could seldomly appear after a later trauma or a serious quarrel or fight with the partner.

We enter into an empathetic dialogue with our counselees and provide them with an approach by evaluating their problems as our own. In fact, the problem is a taboo and an inexplicable secret among spouses so they feel the same distress in front of the physician too. A complete harmony is attained after the dialogue established in the first session. The woman's partner is able to watch her via our closed circuit camera system. And that creates an additional factor of trust.

After the sessions, in phone conversations or via e-mail, we listen to their experiences and the problems they face, and we provide new approaches. This way, they find true support for a problem they had been trying to deal with on their own for years. Together with this trust, they gradually proceed towards the solution of their problem.

Below is the summary of how the approaches used for vaginismus treatment have evolved and developed in time.

Psychoanalytic Approach

One of the first approaches used in vaginismus treatment has been the psychoanalytic approach. According to this approach, vaginismus results from reasons such as fear of castration or penis jealousy. Therefore, the resolution of subconscious conflicts has been targeted in treatment.

Behaviorist Approach

One of the traditional approaches used in the treatment of vaginismus is the behaviorist approach. In this approach, which is based on a completely different perspective compared to the psychoanalytic approach, is grounded on the view that believes that sexual behaviors are learned behaviors and that sexual dysfunctions are based on wrong learnings. Therefore, the treatment emphasizes on the things that have been wrongly learned, and the focal point is the patient with vaginismus. In the treatment on the basis of this viewpoint, deep muscle relaxation and systematic desensitization methods based on learning rules are utilized.

Masters & Johnson Approach

Also based on a behaviorist viewpoint but different from psychoanalytic and other behaviorist approaches, Masters and Johnson have suggested a therapy approach that focuses on the couple and the relationship between the spouses. One of the most important features of this treatment approach is that it comprises common techniques that can be used for all functional disorders, as well as specific techniques for different dysfunctions. The treatment emphasizes on sexual education, communication types between spouses, and the changing of the wrong behavior that cause the occurrence or continuance of vaginismus, and it also involves homework.

Modern Approaches

One of the changes offered in modern approaches has been about the application type of the therapy. For instance, in the approach of Masters and Johnson, the treatment is carried out by two therapists, one male and one female. Certainly there are many benefits of such an application. However, as most treatment centers that work on sexual dysfunctions do not have the possibility to use two therapists, the treatment is carried out by a single therapist. And in various research, it has been put forward that using a one or two therapists during the meetings is not a factor in terms of the treatment's success. Hence, the general practice in modern approaches is having one therapist for the treatment.

Another change in the application style is regarding the frequency of the meetings. In Masters and Johnson's approach, the couple is met every day. Whereas the general practice in modern approaches is to have meetings once or twice a week. In their studies, in which they compared daily therapies with therapies done once or twice a week, Clement and Schmidt have also pointed out that less frequent therapies are more successful. (*Note: As you will be reading in future pages, in Turkey, the patient's wish to do the homework is reduced when the treatment duration is prolonged, and the possibility that they will leave the treatment increases. And this is proof that treatment options may vary according to culture. In the therapy he applies, the therapist has to take into consideration the cultural differences*).

One of the most important differences between the Masters and Johnson approach and modern therapy approaches is that the requirement for both spouses to attend the meetings has been removed. Even though the general approach in treatment is for spouses to attend the meetings together, the husband may not need to attend all meetings if there are no important relationship and communication problems between spouses, if homeworks are done regularly, and if the imposed prohibitions are followed. The important thing regarding the treatment is that the man sustains cooperation with the woman, even if he does not attend all meetings. Again, some researches have investigated to see whether the gender of the therapist and the gender of the patient being the same was a factor in the success of the treatment or not. In general, such research have come to the conclusion that the gender of the therapist and the gender of the patient being same or different did not have any importance in terms of treatment. (*Note: The important thing is the therapist's experience level*).

In modern approaches, contrary to Masters and Johnson's approach, it is thought that treatment needs to be multifaceted and   reintegrative, depending on the factors that play a role in the occurrence or continuation of vaginismus. In other words, an eclectic approach is utilized in modern sexual treatments. For instance, Havvton has applied behaviorist and cognitive therapy methods in the treatment of sexual dysfunctions, whereas Kaplan joins behaviorist and psychoanalytic therapy methods. Another eclectic approach that could be used in the treatment of sexual functionality disorders is the usage of cognitive and Gestalt Therapy methods together.

And in my own approach, I am using *hypnotherapy together with cognitive and behaviorist methods.*

I believe that hypnotherapy can be used in vaginismus treatment as a current approach, and that hypnotherapy is able to provide success in terms of mechanics and also pleasure, while other methods provide only mechanical solutions. Moreover, hypnotherapy is able to create faster solutions for problems in vaginismus.

Hypnotherapy in vaginismus plays active role in,
1. Increasing belief in success,
2. Supporting the ego,
3. Replacing contractions with relaxation,
4. Creating awareness in the patient that she has control over her body,
5. Preparing the mind with simulation (i.e. visualization) for both homework and also for the experience.

THE MAIN PROBLEM IN VAGINISMUS IS THE MEANING ASCRIBED TO THE EMOTIONS AND TO THE SITUATION

When we talk about vaginismus, it is possible to formulate it according to the causes that create the problems,
1. Cognitive
2. Behavioral
3. Dynamic
4. Existentialist

While performing vaginismus treatment, using this formulation while working according to the causes will bring along a systematic study.

Fine, but is that all?

The result from my studies is that all these are visual causes. There is also a backstage, a hidden side to everything…

The meanings ascribed to the emotions and the situation. Among the vaginismus patients, there are physicians, gynecologists, nurses, midwives, and psychologists. The vaginismus patients with such professions know many things to the finest details due to their occupations. But in their own words, "Knowing doesn't provide solution." They also say, "Despite the fact that I know what is what, what needs to be done, that something can go in there, and although I have performed genital applications with my patients, I can't control my will."

Yes, the creator of the problem is the subconscious system, and at the moment of intercourse, the subconscious system is not accepting the conscious system's experiences and knowledge.

So, how can that happen?

The meanings, miscoded by emotions and ascribed to the moment of intercourse, are the primary triggers for the problem. According to our factory settings at birth, intercourse is essential for reproduction and for the continuance of the bloodline, and this is fine-tuned to the tiniest detail with the organs, the nervous system and hormones.

But we see that emotions and the meanings ascribed to them can be altered during the childhood and adolescence period, when the person is learning curiously. Intercourse, which is natural and evolutionary, becomes impossible as the negative emotions and the ascribed meanings show their effects on the subconscious, thus restructuring the system.

And this is actually the best indicator which shows us that the emotions and ascribed meanings can alter the subconscious in contrast with evolution.

A patient of mine was a technical draftsman and when his daughter reached puberty, he had sat her down and informed her by drawing up the genital organs. But his daughter was sitting across from me with vaginismus when she got married. Therefore, it would be very accurate to say, "It will be much more beneficial for a correct sexual life if parents would inform their children with love, without inflicting fright, in a language that can be understood at the child's age, and in a healthy communication while teaching sexuality." But as I have emphasized earlier, it is not just the absence or wrongness of sexual education that creates the problem. Such absence and wrongness only covers a small portion of patients diagnosed with vaginismus, and simply providing this group with information could bring the solution. According to my studies, I could say that this group is about ten percent of patients who apply with vaginismus diagnosis.

The remaining ninety percent suffer, in degrees varying from light to severe, a the process where the willpower becomes disabled and where involuntary contractions, withdrawals and repulsions are seen in addition to symptoms of panic attack.

As an interesting metaphor, the vaginismus patient could define the penis penetrating the vagina as, "You know how you try to touch your pupil and you flinch and your eyelids close automatically…that is exactly how I feel." This metaphor is the best example that defines the patient's subconscious reflex arc in vaginismus. It is the message that says, "I want it in my conscious but I react unwillingly."

In fact, the wording above presents the reason why problems are frequently observed during the *behavioral treatments* that externalize the mind.

There are four main factors in The Dr. Ulusoy Method for Vaginismus Treatment.
1. Psychoeducation
2. Cognitive Approach
3. Behavioral Treatment
4. Problem-driven use of Hypnotherapy

This is how it offers the best and fastest results. As observed in my own studies, and as I have presented during the European Hypnosis Congress, the result may be obtained in twenty-four hours on average after starting the treatment. At this point, of course it is necessary to be reminded that the classical treatment has a treatment protocol that lasts twelve weeks (Three months) with weekly meetings. There is a serious difference when we compare the durations of both treatments. In addition, during the classical treatment, sometimes the homeworks are not done by the patient, or she moves away from treatment because it lasts so long, or she may do everything but she still may not be successful at the time of intercourse. These are the visible risks of classical treatment.

If we think of this problem, which is created by the vaginismus patients unwillingly and unwittingly, in terms of reverse engineering, it would be correct to say, "If we know that *the emotions and the meanings ascribed to events are able to alter the subconscious,* we could use the same mechanism to make it possible to positively develop the subconscious on different subjects." It is possible to use hypnotherapy to use this mechanism to mature and to motivate a person, to provide her adaptation to life, and to help her improve in creating new emotional paths.

SUGGESTIONS FOR VAGINISMUS PATIENTS

Sometimes we receive questions such as, "There are some suggestions in forums for using fingers, devices, candles, fruits and different types of oil. How true are these?"

Saying, "I succeeded, you should try these too," is the worst thing a vaginismus patient can do to another vaginismus patient.

See, I have solved the problems of 146 people by providing free support on the internet during the years 2005 and 2006. But there were 1460 people in the group. So, only ten percent of the vaginismus cases that we could call simple ones were able to solve the problem with education. Later I stopped this service because,

1. While treating the 146 people, you may cause the remaining 1314 persons to waste their time and to fall into despair. Time is very valuable in vaginismus. It requires treatment in a short time with the correct approach. Besides, you will obstructing her future treatment by creating the idea, "I tried too, but I couldn't succeed. I am a difficult patient," in the minds of those who have not been healed. In short, the treatment becomes worse than the disease.

   As for the cured patients; you may have been healed but everyone's vaginismus is different, it is not the same. Patients' anatomies, characters are different. If you simplify the procedures in your treatments and say, "I did this and that, you should do it too and it will be gone," you will be unwillingly hurting your fellow patients.

   I had such a patient who disregarded the hypnotic suggestions she had received and who acted as if she had solved the problem simply with a device. She suggested the same device to a friend of hers who had the same problem. Her friend used the device but could not have intercourse. This woman came to me later for treatment and we had serious problems with her because she had wrongly exercised by herself. Please do not hurt your fellow patients.

2. It is simply not right to suggest products that do not conform to the nature of the vagina.

3. There is a serious situation that we call *vagal stimulus*. In the applications done at home by oneself -with the suggestions of healed patients- serious

problems may occur if vagal stimuli are activated. Syncope (Sudden drop in blood pressure and fainting) may be observed.

4. In the applications at home, albeit rarely, there could be problems at the hymen. If it is deformed and starts bleeding, and if the patient cannot stop the bleeding on her own, this would also be a serious problem.

Those, who have been treated and healed, and who give advice to others for applying the same things, and those who rely on healed patients for the cure, please read my words carefully and take note.

The best thing healed patients can do is to provide moral support to other vaginismus patients and to support them in their treatment. Other than this, telling them to do this or that may cause serious damage as I have stated above.

IS IT CORRECT TO CLASSIFY VAGINISMUS CASES ACCORDING TO DIFFICULTY?

Recently, some of our patients that call us start their words with, "I saw a classification online and I seem to be a simple (or difficult) case…"

This is a totally wrong perspective because of the following reasons.

1. I have mostly worked with patients that had applied to many places but were unable to be cured, that were evaluated as difficult patients. I observed that these patients were also healed in a short time. Therefore, the difficultness or easiness depends on the method of the therapist.

2. I saw that it is not possible to classify such cases as easy or difficult before the treatment.

3. The easiness or difficultness of the case depends on the therapist's perspective and his treatment approach. If the appropriate treatment for the patient is applied, the case is a simple one. Otherwise it is difficult.

4. The case being truly difficult or easy is in parallel with the patient's character patterns. And these patterns are not obvious before starting face-to-face work with the patient. The therapist needs to have enough experience to solve the character-based resistances that will come up during the treatment.

5. One should know that cases that seem to be easy may prove to be difficult and vice versa. Therefore, difficulty-based classification in vaginismus cases is not correct. Each applying case is an unknown. Vaginismus is solved step by step with feedbacks. So, each case is simple with the therapist's appropriate approach. Frankly, if the case cannot be solved, it is not because of the case being difficult but because of the therapist's wrong approach to the patient, or due to his lack of knowledge, skills or experience. Therefore, specifically tailor-made, atheoretical (M. Erickson) approaches are necessary for each and every patient. And this means that therapists, who have worked on many cases, who have gained experience and who have improved themselves in this field, are required.

6. The case's difficulty-based classification causes the patient to unintentionally fall into stereotypes. For instance, she will be left in the question, "If it was so easy, why is the process so long. Why can't it be solved yet?" Or if an easy case is classified as a difficult case, the treatment process could be driven into a deadlock.

Each case of vaginismus is unique because of the differences in character patterns.

If you do not take this into consideration and take the standard behaviorist approach as in classical approaches, you will see cases that cannot be solved. For this reason, there are many cases in Turkey that have been treated in various places but that have remained unhealed.

I can describe this as the following; you know how they give the baby a toy bucket with a star, a circle, a triangle and a square hole, and the baby tries to put the geometrical toys in his hands into those holes… If your treatment type is just classical and behaviorist, it will be like trying to put the wrong shapes into the wrong hole. And this complicates the problem even further, rather than solving it.

Of course, I would also like to remind you that the patient's willingness and compatibility with the treatment, as well as her involvement in the process until the end of the treatment is also necessary.

It is not correct to make a difficulty-based classification in vaginismus treatment!

CLASSIFICATION OF VAGINISMUS PATIENTS

(Dr. Ulusoy - 2008)

1. Those who cannot touch the labia majora or labia minora, or in between (Outer genitalia).
2. Those who can touch the outer genital area but not inside the vagina.
3. Those who can touch the outer genitalia and the vagina and can direct fingers inside, but who cannot have the penis experience.
4. Those who are in one of the three groups mentioned above and who do not have contractions, but who cannot allow the penis inside (Those with hip problems, breathing control problems or with problems of transferring of authority).
5. Those who are in one of the first three groups mentioned above and who have internal or external contractions ranging from minor to severe, and who cannot take in the penis.

As seen, various categories appear when we talk about vaginismus. Moreover the factors listed below also have effect on the woman at different proportions, so the vaginismus illness almost resembles an ivy.

1. The woman's own character patterns (i.e. panic attack, obsession, perfectionist structure, phobic and afraid of everything…).
2. Lack of sexual education and knowledge.
3. Physical differences between man and woman.
4. Cognitive, behavioral, dynamic and existentialistic factors.

Therefore, the vaginismus treatment should be planned by taking into consideration all these details.

At the same time, the *woman-man-therapist* trivet should be on solid ground. If one of the legs of the trivet is problematic, disruptions in the treatment will be inevitable.

A PARADOX IN VAGINISMUS

Some vaginismus patients may have fears that are brought by their personality structure and that have spread all around. For instance, fear of elevators, of driving, of having injections, fear of the dark, of insects or animals, etc. This structure could also be a sign which shows that the etiopathogenesis (creation mechanism) of vaginismus could be resulting from interactions with the family or with the environment during childhood or puberty. While the dough of our personality is shaped during those years, some unpleasant or disturbing substances may have been mixed in the dough.

While one of the two sisters living in the same house has vaginismus, the other may have comfortable relationships. And this shows us that the woman's character patterns are more influential in vaginismus, rather than being affected by the same setting and environment.

Let's provide an anecdote: One day, my patient's husband said, "My wife is scared a lot. She can't even feed the fish at home." The first things that came to my mind were red goldish and I asked, "What type of fish do you have at home?" and I found out that they had two piranhas in the fish tank. ☺

Some vaginismus patients say that they have had injections, endoscopic stomach examinations, surgical interventions and that they have endured many things but that they just could not overcome this thing.

Another vaginismus patient group says, "I can't have intercourse with my partner but I tried other relationships with him -oral and anal- to have other kinds of pleasure. I am able to take the penis from the back."

A different vaginismus patient group says that they can allow finger penetration or any other object but not the penis (Vaginismus classification – Dr. Ulusoy).

When we look at the last three groups, we see that there are cases, in which the woman is able to take in the endoscopic examination hose from the mouth, which can have anal intercourse but which cannot take the penis inside. In such cases, the vaginismus woman askes in disbelief, "Why not? Isn't that place something like the anus?"

Well, after all, the mouth and the esophagus were created for the eating function, and the anus was created appropriate for defecation. And the vagina was created for intercourse, perfectly for the penetration of the penis.

The reason why it cannot penetrate is not mechanical!

It is the result of the emotional meaning one ascribes to the vagina over time…

The fact that it seems to be mechanical is caused by physicians' focusing on the visible part -the bodily reactions- instead of focusing on the reason. And many patients think this way, too. So when they apply to various places and cannot be cured, they say, "I went everywhere but it was not cured, I could not succeed," and blame themselves, rather than looking at the process and method of their treatment. The *Karagöz and Hacivat²* shadow play is a reflection we watch on the screen, and the treatments that see things solely as mechanical and that focus on working on the vagina during vaginismus treatment are only fighting shadows; whereas the actual place of treatment is where the puppet master is, and that is the subconscious.

And here, for this reason, we once again repeat the sentence that we keep on saying, "Vaginismus is an illness in which the mental and emotional state manifests physical symptoms, and its treatment should be planned accordingly."

If one tries to remove the emotional reflex arcs with deficient treatments that ignore the mind and solely target the vagina, either the treatment remains unsuccessful, or it proves successful but the reflex arcs revive in later times, causing the vaginismus to resurface once again. Or there could be problems about having pleasure after such treatment.

Finally, let's end this part by touching upon the other two paradoxes seen in vaginismus.

1. The fact that some vaginismus patients can easily have examinations, mostly cause their gynecologists to tell them that they do not have vaginismus. But vaginismus is not an illness that can be diagnosed by examination but by the patient conveying her experiences at the time of intercourse.

2. The foreign vaginismus patients, referred to in foreign literature as *secondary vaginismus*, have contractions and closures in the lower 1/3 of vaginal parts. And treatments, such as expansion works or botox applications, are carried out mechanically to remove this contraction. On the other hand, in the primary vaginismus seen in Turks, the vagina is loose. Anything can go inside but there are mind-body related reactions that do not allow the penetration of the penis.

---

(2) **TN:** Karagöz and Hacivat are the lead characters of the traditional Turkish shadow play, popularized during the Ottoman period and then spread to most nation states that comprised the Ottoman Empire.

WHY IS IT THAT COUPLES SEEK VAGINISMUS TREATMENT AFTER LONG YEARS OF MARRIAGE?

When we observe patients coming in for vaginismus treatment, we see that the number of those who have success and those who apply for treatment shortly after getting married is not so great. We see that there are vaginismus patients who wait from one to thirty years, or who cannot have not had success in their treatments. Why is that so?

1. Many couples cannot understand the situation when they are not able to have their first night experience. There are fears, contractions, withdrawals, crying jags, etc. Months and years go by without being able to identify the problem.

2. There are those who identify the situation but who think it will pass in time if they wait.

3. There are those who think they can solve it on their own, trying to find support in books, on the internet and in forum pages. These women do not realize that those who are able to solve the problem on their own are the ten percent minority with simple vaginismus. They also disregard the fact that every vaginismus is different and that there are different physical, emotional and personality structures for each individual. So they lose time and sometimes they deepen the problem with wrong suggestions and applications.

4. Once they decide to have treatment, then the efficiency of the treatment comes into prominence. Unfortunately, problems occur in choices made without considering the efficiency of the treatment. The ratio of those who apply to one, two, three, five or even more places but who cannot be treated is about thirty percent (According to a survey with 5900 women. Please see the survey section at the end).

5. Time can also be wasted with wrong applications caused by the mistakes of the physician or in the therapy process, which we call iatrogenic. (Hymen operations, botox applications, unproven therapy approaches under anesthesia or with epidural, sending the patient home with a prescription, or therapists who say they will absolutely provide the cure but who cannot…are all disheartening.)

6. Time is also lost when the couple does not try to solve the vaginismus problem but submits to the pressure from their surroundings and tries to have a baby with in vitro fertilization.
7. After some time, a minority of men accept the situation as it is, or they build a secret life for themselves outside the home, or they get divorced.
8. After a certain period of time, the couple that experiences all the items above starts to think that the problem is without a cure and ignores it.

We sadly observe that the mistakes we listed in the above eight items are repeated by many vaginismus couples.

VAGINISMUS AND CONVERSION

Vaginismus is not an illness on its own. Even if it seems like a problem originated in the lower vaginal muscles, the vagina is loose in the vaginismus seen in Turkish women. The entire problem is the mental and physical panic attack symptoms that surface at the moment of intercourse. These symptoms mostly become uncontrollable. As a matter of fact, vaginismus mostly comes together with symptoms of panic attack. It can also be together with conversion, too.

A patient we worked on had had classical treatment for ten months with two meetings a week. She hardly performed the exercises regarding the vagina but the experience did not happen. Years followed each other and seven years passed by. Seizures and contraction episodes, which we define as conversive, were added to the problem in environments where she had fear, insecurity, and felt herself in danger or in distress.

During our preliminary meeting with this patient, she developed conversive episodes triggered by seizures and contractions accompanied by dizziness. She had five consecutive episodes during this first meeting. We laid the patient on her back, to the Trendelenburg position (On her back, head lower and feet higher) and gave her a supportive talk to take her out of the seizure.

In the emergency rooms, such conversive patients are given diazepam and the patient goes through the episode in a sleep state. But according to S. Grof, such episodes are emotional crises. If the patient can be taken out of the seizure by talking and supporting, it will serve as a healing factor for the patient.

The seizure experienced by our patient was evaluated as a different state of consciousness that provided escape and also as an emotional crisis, so she was supported with suggestions each time. Without the usage of any sedative medicine, the situation was taken under control after the first hour and the treatment was resumed.

With her emotional crisis and with my supportive approach, the patient entered an inner healing process. Throughout the day, the mechanical and hypnotherapy exercises of our three-stage treatment were completed without problems and she was given a one-day rest. The next morning, I supported her once again with suggestions and led the couple toward intercourse.

If there had been any deficiencies in the healing process of her emotional crisis or in my hypnotherapy method, our patient could have had a conversive episode during the intercourse as an act of avoidance.

A short while later, we received the news that our patient had had a smooth intercourse experience.

During this process, the role of our hypnotherapy studies and our correct directing of the emotional crisis by revealing the inner healing effect of the mind without using sedatives was great.

Based on this case, we once again verified the necessity of not viewing the problem in vaginismus patients solely as mechanical, and of working on the mind with hypnotherapy.

ANESTHESIA, SUBCONSCIOUS AND VAGINISMUS

We know that the conscious is deactivated under anesthesia. Since the conscious is disabled, it cannot be aware of the events around. Moreover, the feelings of pain and ache are blocked, and a deep relaxation occurs in the body.

So, what does the subconscious do during this time?

Even if the conscious is deactivated, the subconscious is scanning both its inner system and also the environment by using the five senses and the system beyond the senses. It is evaluating the incoming data and processing them.

There has been success in the classical (Pavlovian) conditioning experiments done under anesthesia. And this shows that the subconscious is able to receive classical conditioning suggestions beyond the conscious.

Another point I would like to emphasize is some doctors' iatrogenic suggestions and experiments for the vaginismus patient to have intercourse under anesthesia. In some cases I have worked on, I have heard stories of patients having tried such an experience. Epidural or anesthesia have been wrongly administered and the man has been offered intercourse with the women in such state.

The words of the men were interesting, "While completely under anesthesia, her legs closed and she convulsed when I approached to have intercourse."

How does that happen? Even if the conscious is by-passed with anesthetic substances, the subconscious is able to perceive the thing that it fears and to react. Vaginismus is not actually a problem concerning the vagina. Vaginismus is a total mental illness of the subconscious. And the treatment should primarily be founded on the subconscious.

In such cases, unfortunately, the intercourse that is meant to be experienced under anesthesia is perceived by the subconscious as molestation and rape, thus further complicating the problem. Many more difficulties arise while working with such cases when compared to others.

IS THE VAGINISMUS WOMAN SPOILED?

Consultee: I have the same problem; I've been married for eleven months. I haven't been with my husband since eleven months. I am scared and worried, I think that it will hurt and that is why it scares me even to try. So our marriage is going worse each day. We constantly argue with my husband. Even if the topic of the argument isn't this, I think that the actual source of every argument is this problem. I had not been able to take my husband to the physician because he thought that I was just acting spoilt and that it had nothing to do with a doctor. But finally I managed to persuade him. I don't want my marriage to end because of an unexperienced event. After all, we fell in love and got married…

Dr. Ulusoy: Ah, the men! When will they understand that you ladies are not spoiled or just being whimsical, and that you have a problem at the subconscious level? When will they support you? No woman can say, "No" to an intercourse she desires just for the sake of acting spoiled or caprice. She especially is unable to control her body and put it in a state where it has contractions at the legs, tension in the hands, or where it pushes the partner away, or has crying spells.

The partners of women with vaginismus should absolutely know that a sarcastic, blaming attitude will be like adding fuel to the flames. They should support their partners at every step, love and respect them, and always keep alive the thrill of their first love. Vaginismus women are like paper dolls, they require more care… They will always repay you exceedingly for the attention you give them. The men should not support the treatment with the goal of having children or for the intercourse to take place, but they should remain by their spouse in order to have a lifetime of happy sexuality with them.

Dear men, take another look at your spouse, look again, look closer… If you want to have a happy sex life for the rest of your life, go on and say nice things to her. I bet you have neglected your wife for a long time… When was the last time you bought her flowers? When was the last time you remembered a special day?

Women are like *everblooming roses*. When you take one step toward them, you will see that they will come running with joy. Why do you spare your nice words when it is so easy to please them? Why? When was the last time you embraced her sincerely? When did she last lay her head on your shoulder? When was the last time you thanked her for something ordinary that she did? When was the last time you gave her a kiss when you left in the morning or returned home in the evening? When did you last show compassion instead of getting mad when she was at fault; when did you forgive her?

Come on my fellow men, this is the time to take action, take small steps… Let the everblooming roses blossom every season, let them give us comfort with their beauty and their scents…

DOES YOUR SPOUSE SUPPORT YOU?

Consultee: Yes, when I read your latest post in the group, I realized that the reasons of my vaginismus are integrated with my husband's indifference… The unconcernedness of my man, the way he leads a life like a robot caught in the flow of life… The way he ignores me… He goes on with his life as if he was content with it or as if he does not care at all. I am very comfortable while working with vaginal expanders by myself. But when I'm with him, something comes over me. A man who fights for nothing… I am starting to think that I am resisting because I am pissed off with his insensitivity and circumvention…

Dr. Ulusoy: You are obviously being neglected and you are doing everything on your own… What can you do to express yourself, to prove to himself, to say that you are there? Think about it and trust your inner mind with this…

Sex is a need; you should not keep yourself away from this need whether you love your husband or not. You can hate him, accuse him of insensitivity; this is natural. But when you need to experience sex, don't think of it as an attitude against your husband or as a reward for him. Have sex because you want to, so you can feel the pleasure of it. You can almost use him for your sexuality. And don't be surprised if he starts to change in time and takes some steps. While having the relationship, keep a broad imagination and visualize that you are having sex with the prince in your dreams. Be the winning side. Just use him and let him go. Assume the same indifferent attitude after having sex. What do you say; is it worth a try?

Another Consultee: I congratulate you very very much for your words and thoughts. For telling us all about this as bare facts and for giving us this advice, as a man yourself... Actually, I used to be like that lady for many years, seven years. I always thought I was guilty, the one with the problem, so I tried to do everything I could to make him happy in every sense, almost breaking my soul for him. But then I saw that the other party, my husband, was very happy with this and he was using this. I told myself to stop, enough, don't let the years pass by this way. "Let it break if it has to," I said to myself, "Live for yourself from now on." Sex? I'm using him whenever I feel like it... Then, with the same indifferent attitude, I make him feel that I have used him for sex... In fact, just the other day, he asked me during foreplay, "Did you really have an orgasm or are you just acting to comfort me?" And I said, "Those times have past. If I like it, I live it to the fullest. If not, I'll tell you to stop and tell you openly."

I think all women should be frank about this; they should not make compromises from their personality. I am thirty-four years old and I have never had intercourse with my husband. But I have realized that I am not the one with all the problems, he has them too. Because once, two months ago, I was able to have intercourse with someone I knew from the past. Without medicine, narcosis, sedatives or antidepressants... So apparently it was possible. It just needed some effort, trust and patience. Of course my husband does not know this but my self-confidence as a woman has increased so much that I am able to leave everything behind just like that. And he is aware of this so he shows me more interest, just as you said...

Mr. Murat, I applaud you for your candor and for honestly touching upon this point as a man. Really, there are so few people, men, who would admit this... No matter what profession they are in... This shows how much you at peace with yourself and that you are wholeheartedly trying to help women like us. I wish you continued success...

I would very much appreciate it if you could allow other women to see my letter.

Dr. Ulusoy: Nevertheless, when there is an existing family order, infidelity should not be tolerated.

SEX LIFE AND VAGINISMUS

Contrary to popular belief, most women with vaginismus are able to reach sexual pleasure and satisfaction with other ways. Of course, the couples should not be blaming each other after every unsuccessful penis-vagina intercourse trial. If couples know that they will be successful when they accept the situation and find the right method when the time comes, they are able to have much more pleasure out of sex when compared to other couples. The woman is able to reach satisfaction in their togetherness that they continue with sensual-tactile and other representing systems, and with their sex games.

Rarely, there are also women who do not want to have intercourse due to lack of sexual desire. Such situations may be wrongly evaluated as vaginismus by couples. Women are provided with training on orgasm and sex life with hypnotherapy. With the work done together, orgasm can be taught in two-hour therapies for those who have had at least one orgasm before, and in four to six-hour therapies for women who have never experienced orgasm. If there are no hormonal imbalances, of course...

By refraining from negativities such as, "Oh, dear! I have vaginismus... My life is done; it's all over. I had no success from therapy either," you can reach the pleasure and satisfaction of sex with love games, romance, with sex games and approaches. This point that you will experience in sex, will send messages to your subconscious for your vaginismus to be solved more easily.

Vaginismus is not an obstacle for sex! Don't let it become one. In return for the woman's pleasure and satisfaction, the man also wants to reach orgasm and to ejaculate. Therefore, the woman needs to be more active in such relationships, to remove her taboos about sex and experiments, and to know how to give her spouse an orgasm. It will be appropriate for the woman to use her hands during sex, to almost feel and sense her spouse's body, as a blind person would feel her hands. The same approach is valid for the man, too. In order for him to bring his wife to vaginal orgasm, love games, sensual approaches, kissing and caressing of the body and the genital structure, and stimulation of the clitoris with hands and tongue are essential. The pleasure of the couples could be enhanced with the usage of oral structures. It is recommended that couples read related books and sex life manuals together.

VAGINISMUS AND PREGNANCY

"My husband and I had begun taking support from a psychologist but nothing was achieved. One day, during one of our trials, my husband ejaculated on my vagina. I mean, he never penetrated, just ejaculated over it and I got pregnant! When we went to the physician, he did not believe us and wanted to examine me. He told me that such thing was impossible, and I told him that it was also impossible for him to examine me ☺ and that I wanted to have an abortion. And, hold on to your hat; I was pregnant but I was also still a virgin! So, the doctor also removed my hymen during the abortion. He had never heard of such a case before he met me, nor did he even know about vaginismus!"

"Hello, Mr. Murat. I have been following the messages. I decided to write since I was also a vaginismus patient (Once upon a time) who had a child. I have been married for six years and I have a two-year-old child. I have overcome this illness just two days ago. Thanks to Mr. Murat, of course. I had gone to a psychiatrist in Istanbul earlier, and during that treatment, my husband ejaculated in our intercourse trials and I got pregnant, I was so surprised. We were baffled at how it could happen like that. And we could never try intercourse again, anyway. I got pregnant without having penetration, intercourse, and I know there are a lot of people like me. Anyway, I reached Mr. Murat through a friend of mine and I overcame this menace fear in my mind with hypnosis. We were successful at the end of the third session. My husband and I are very happy…should we go on a second honeymoon or what? Thanks again Mr. Murat. Nirvana…"

Dr. Ulusoy: Other than artificial insemination, in some methods that offer single-session solutions, painkillers, muscle relaxants, sedatives and hip baths are advised. Or, pregnancy could be seen by the accidental entrance of the sperms into the vagina during epidural anesthetics, botox or inadequate therapies. Those who apply such methods do so for one time, even if they don't completely remember it afterwards. What happens later? As the situation continues in the subconscious, there has been no cure and they still cannot have intercourse. The money they have spent aside, their moral collapse is more serious…

For this reason, we especially prefer hypnotherapy, subconscious approaches and mental maneuvers in vaginismus. We go to the source of the problem and solve it there…

While working at the Medical Faculty Gynecology Polyclinic, there was an eighteen-year-old girl who had not had her periods for four months and she was trying to find out the reason. In the ultrasound we performed, we detected a four-month pregnancy. The girl thought we were joking and said, "But it's impossible, my partner never ejaculated inside me..."

Even if your partner does not ejaculate inside you, he can impregnate you while ejaculating outside the vagina. And, if the penis has entered the vagina but not ejaculated inside, various secretions are released from the penis during intercourse before the actual sperm-containing semen. Sometimes, there is sperm, even if very few, in these secretions and they will leave you impregnated. Therefore, we don't find odd those who become pregnant while having vaginismus, and we don't advice ejaculating outside as a pregnancy prevention method...

STATE OF MIND OF THE VAGINISMUS MAN

We looked at vaginismus as the woman's problem but we should also give ear to the words of a man with a vaginismus wife.

If your wife has vaginismus,
1. Every now and then, you get the feeling that she doesn't love you and it makes you feel devastated.
2. Your dreams of having a child gradually disappear. You become unable to look at small children. It hurts to play with your friends' kids. Even the diaper commercials are enough to upset you.
3. You start developing a great loss of sexual desire. You even become unable to masturbate.
4. You have lost all hope for the solving of this situation which has not been solved for three years. Hence, you are unable to contribute to your wife's efforts.
5. You blame yourself, saying, "If she hadn't married me, maybe she wouldn't be in this situation. She would have been happy."
6. Although you love her more than anything, you want her to leave you and build a happy home. You even try to push her away from yourself.
7. You start seeing her as your daughter due to the age gap.

8. When you are really drunk, you have fantasies of cheating on her just to prove your manhood. But you hate yourself the next day for thinking that.
9. Your unhappiness at home reflects to work. You become inefficient even if you work a lot.
10. Alcohol has become your best friend. You drink almost every day, to the point of passing out.
11. You want to die but you can't, because you don't want to upset those who love you.
12. Everyone thinks you are cheerful. But you cry secretly.
13. You block people from commenting on your confessions because you know that no help or comment will be helpful.
14. Your keyboard has become wet while typing your confessions.

A vaginismus man…

STATE OF MIND OF THE VAGINISMUS WOMAN

"This is hard until you get over it, I guess. Once you do, maybe it will be a week before you even forget having such a problem. But those who experience it are still struggling inside that vortex. I have been having classical treatment for a month. I've come quite a way; even I am surprised with the distance I have covered with finger exercises. But I guess I will not be able to believe that I can do it until the final day. Vaginismus is like learning to swim, to ride a bicycle. Once you gather your courage and hit the pedals, you are able to do it after seeing that you don't fall, that you speed up. But there, we need wind to revive this belief. The air feels so droughty nowadays… There is no more wind from my right or from my left… What I'm trying to say is that I am solving the problem mechanically, yes, but I have been feeling very bad for the last week because I am in depression. I just don't want to talk to anyone, I just want to stay in my room and sleep. I eat only enough to keep me alive, I keep on trying to slur life over. For some reason, I feel that it is too late for the successes I have achieved to make me happy. There is a meaningless weariness over me. I stir up trouble for no reason and I cry, I upset my husband and torture myself too. I am even surprised if the meal I cook tastes nice.

You know the story of the ugly duckling…I feel exactly like the ugly duck there. I am about to give up on life. I have lost my health too, I can't sleep, I can't concentrate on work. I am always depressed all the time… People around me keep asking what is bothering me nowadays. How could I tell them? What would happen if I did? I keep asking why this is happening to me. And as I do, I start digging out the past. My old boyfriends… I went through my past with a fine comb. I wondered if one of them did this to me; such silly thoughts I have… I stood up today for just half an hour. I have formed five sentences at most. I am so unhappy I just can't explain, so unhappy…"

VAGINISMUS, BROTHELS AND MEN

How are men affected by going to a brothel in their youth or when they are unable to have sex during marriage?

Men are interested in having their first experience as soon as they enter puberty. How is it done? Can I do it? How long will it last? How many times can I do it? Is mine sufficient in length, width, etc.

When we take a look at it, they are drawing a cartoon of sex life that is far from emotions and totally based on physical structures. But the fact that mental control lies behind physical control is neglected.

Now let's continue with an example from a patient.

A young and newlywed couple, the wife has vaginismus. The man loves his wife very much and he has warm feelings for her, he does not want to harm or hurt her. He has been in brothels many times in the past. He talks with pride, "It used to last so long that it would take an hour before I came. After all, I was paying for it; I liked it to last long. And most of the time, the women begged me to ejaculate."

In this first paragraph of our story, there is a man, who pays for record trials, who wants to satisfy his savage and wild inner sex drives, and who chooses to prolong the intercourse as much as possible so that he can take his money's worth. And on the other hand, there is a service provider far from emotions, who waits for him to penetrate, give the money and go.

The mind builds new physical control constructions with learned, experienced information and remembers this construction -scheme- later in similar conditions and starts the necessary process.

And when our man gets married and tries to have intercourse, he meets a woman whose feelings are prominent -unlike the ones in the brothel- and moreover, who has vaginismus because of her fearful feelings about intercourse.

They immediately came over for treatment. His wife's treatment was completed within twenty-four hours with Dr. Ulusoy HIT and VTT. Just as they were being directed toward intercourse, the man was asked, "Do you have erection problems?"

Bragging, the man said, "No, doctor, I don't. It remains erect for almost an hour, I don't ejaculate easily," with the pride of a lion king.

They were sent to their hotel for the experience and the good news was awaited. The phone rang or a text arrived, "Doctor, I don't know what happened. I can't get it up. I try and it stiffens a bit but just as I try to go in, it softens again."

I call this situation in vaginismus *The Seesaw Effect*, the man hitting bottom when the woman is ready.

The Seesaw Effect depends on many factors including the following.
1. Quick masturbations
2. Anger and rage reactions developed toward the wife during the vaginismus process
3. Blaming the wife
4. Inexperience
5. Stress and anxiety
6. Dynamic structure (Subconsciously perceiving the wife as his mother)
7. Learned experiences

In our story, it is based on learned experiences as listed in article seven. You look and see that the roaring lion has turned into a mewing little kitty…

The Dr. Ulusoy classification of factors influencing the treatment, there is also a treatment offered to the man in this process. A man in this situation may be offered hypnotherapeutic or medical approaches.

"I have trouble understanding," said the man, "What happened now when I had no problems in the past?"

In fact, there was a problem in the past. You learned wrong. You just went there, paid and experienced impulsive pleasures. On top of that, you had more pleasure when the woman asked you to ejaculate already. You thought you were doing the right thing with your mind and logic at the time; you were buying a service and you wanted to make the most of it…

But now, you have your wife with you. You are not buying a service. With your approach, you first need to caress your wife's feelings and then her soul, and you will enter into a different mental and emotional state of consciousness…

From this point of view, we can say that one reason for the *Seesaw Effect* in man is the brothel experience in the past. These experiences may occur as in our story, or sometimes the harsh and problematic approach of the woman at the brothel may cause erectile dysfunction. Besides, the fact that the woman at the brother does not care for personal hygiene or that she mocks or humiliates you for your failure, will also cause you to be adversely effected by this intercourse. Also, as a learned behavior, it may also reflect negatively on your future experiences.

Stress and anxiety factors are also interesting. Usually, performance worries lie beneath sexual inadequacies. One of our patient's husband was a healthcare professional. We prepared our patient but the man had the Seesaw Effect. Although we provided him with the necessary therapeutic and medical support, he could not have an erection. There were no physiological problems with the man. He was saying that he was not having erection problems during their trials at home, and he was underlining the fact that he was also having morning erections. Then he said this, "I'm a doctor, I work at the ER. Whenever there is a problematic case, I feel anxious and disappear so my colleagues can take care of it. I can't stand stress."

After this message, I asked them to have the intercourse at home. "Your wife is ready now; we don't have any problems with her. No matter how much I support you with therapy and medicine for intercourse at a hotel, you will not only fail but you will also lose confidence and trust in yourself. Therefore, I want you to have intercourse at your own home," I said.

He called back a week later and said, "Doctor, apparently there were no problems with me. I had a normal erection and we had a smooth intercourse. Thank you."

In the end, we are not dealing with an illness, but with a patient. It is important for the vaginismus therapist to see the personality structures of the spouses and to be flexible in the treatment, and also to notice character organizations and adapt to them.

COULD I FORCE IT WITH VAGINISMUS?

Unfortunately, men, who do not realize that vaginismus is an illness, think that they could solve the problem by forcing their spouses into intercourse.

I have come across made anecdotes during the passing time.

1. The man, who told his wife to grit her teeth and that they would have intercourse, was unable to have intercourse and his wife later said, "Doctor, I broke my tooth while gritting it."
2. A man had become raged and angry for not being able to have intercourse and he had beat his wife, locking her in a dark room.
3. One man had tied his wife's hands and feet as he tried to force her into intercourse.
4. As the woman was refraining from vaginismus treatment, she had become pregnant when her husband ejaculated outside. But since she did not have any treatment, her fear of examination and her contractions continued so she had been held down by three or four people during examination and labor, trying to probe her.
5. A man had tried to force his wife into intercourse by giving her sedative drugs, applying anesthesia from the waist down and making her drink alcohol.
6. One man had said, "Doctor, you can see how strong and hulky I am. And my wife is so petite, but when we try to have intercourse, she pushes me away with such a force and has such strong convulsions that I can't really explain."

Vaginismus is a treatable illness. Therefore, one should not try forceful intercourse. Such forcing -as they are perceived as molestation at the subconscious level- make the problem even more complicated.

THREE MAIN OPTIONS IN VAGINISMUS TREATMENT

Many vaginismus patients apply to gynecologists, psychotherapists, physicians and to sex therapists. There is a patient group that is added to this patient pool –population– each year. In the last ten years, the number of physicians and therapists dealing with vaginismus has increased gradually. This is a gladsome thing. Nonetheless, paradoxically, the number of patients did not decrease and unfortunately it continues to grow.

The main reason for this situation is the partial inadequacy in the first and second items you will read below. It is for this reason that The Dr. Ulusoy Method, which is an eclectic approach, is meant to overcome the deficiencies in these two treatments. Moreover, the deficient, lacking, inadequate and unproven treatments that I have mentioned under the topic *Unadvised Approaches to Vaginismus* are also responsible for the increase in the patient population.

So, what could be the reason why the number of patients does not decrease while the number of therapists increases?

1. In the treatments, which are carried out with psychoeducation and homework and which we call the classical treatments, some of the patients don't do their homework or they do the homework but are unable to pass to the trial phase. Unfortunately, classical treatments are hopeless when the homeworks are not done, and the sessions need to be paused until the homeworks are completed, or there should be extra sessions in which the undone homework is completed. If a homework cannot be done, at this point, the therapist has to have different treatment options. Apparently, in the trainings provided to sex therapists, they are not taught any extra options that can be applied in case homework is not done. So the sex therapist may be left hopeless.

2. Some patients also face problems with the behaviorist treatments that are believed to solve vaginismus only by taking something into the vagina. While the patient group that we call simple or intermediate vaginismus can benefit from such treatment, upper intermediate and more severe vaginismus patient groups are unable to take an object or a finger into the vagina, because the mind is not ready or because they cannot pass to the

experience phase after performing the behaviorist homework regarding the vagina.

3. In my opinion, the main problems in the vaginismus faced by Turkish women are the mental-based physical reactions displayed during intercourse. I have evaluated previous cases and I had e-mail correspondences with more than five thousand patients in order to overcome the deficiencies in the first two options above. During this process, I have come across three main structures. *Psychoeducation, Work/Exercise on the vagina, Mind-Body relaxation techniques with suggestion.*

In this context, vaginismus treatment has been restructured and it has been divided into three phases that last approximately twenty-four hours. A therapy model that lasts a total of three or four hours has been developed and it has been presented as a new model in vaginismus treatment during the 12th ESH Istanbul Congress. The majority of our patients become ready for intercourse on the same night. But as a principle, I prefer to have them rest for a night before I talk to them again the next morning and direct them toward intercourse.

Dr. Ulusoy Method in vaginismus treatment eclectically utilizes three separate therapy models that are hypnotherapy, cognitive therapy, and behaviorist therapy. This way, the problem is approached more comprehensively, seeing the reasons that lead the patient to failure in the first two options, and taking them under the scope of the treatment.

Dr. Ulusoy Method II is a hypnosis-based method in vaginismus treatment that allows intercourse within the same day with a three-phase and three-hour work.

In this treatment, *a formulated problem-driven approach + psychoeducation with mirror neuron activation + hypnosis* is utilized. The formulated problem-driven therapy is an eclectic, integrative and gradual treatment, in which the model regarding the relationship is taught, which provides mind-body relaxation by removing contraction, which includes preparation for the relationship model, biofeedback and mindfulness, and where behavioral education and treatment with Holotropic Breathwork applications are applied.

The treatment is directed toward education and creating neuroplasticity in the brain/mind.

The shortness of the treatment duration is due to the work done on the

Psoas Muscle Group, which is the main factor in vaginismus and which I have defined for the first time worldwide.

Other treatments work on the pelvic floor muscles with Kegel Exercises. But in vaginismus, the vagina is loose and vaginismus has nothing to do with pelvic floor muscles. Therefore, other treatments last relatively longer.

UNADVISED APPROACHES TO VAGINISMUS

1. **Removal of the hymen.** There are cases in which vaginismus continues despite the operation on the hymen. The problem is not with the hymen but in the mind. Problems regarding the hymen are rare.
2. **Sexual intercourse under the influence of epidural or general anesthesia.** The subconscious may evaluate this approach as rape. In two cases, the patients said that they were incapacitated from the waist down but when the time came and they tried to take the penis inside, their legs contracted anyway. Another one said, "Doctor, my wife was anesthetized, she was asleep and I entered the room. As I was trying to place my penis into the vagina for intercourse, my wife had convulsions even under anesthesia." In result, although operations can be carried out with hypnoanesthesia and without anesthetic substance if the subconscious is convinced, but the subconscious may produce more reactions when forced into intercourse without being convinced.
3. **Using only anesthetic pomades, sprays and lubricants.** The effect of these drugs on their own is limited. Numbing pomades may be used for short periods if there is a problem with the hymen.
4. **Drugging the woman with medicine or alcohol.** There are women who have become drunk with alcohol but who convulse even more. The problem is in the subconscious. While alcohol disables the conscious, it further activates the subconscious, so using alcohol does not solve the problem.
5. **Taking medication.** Drugs do not solve subconscious problems.
6. **Taking anti-depression or anti-anxiety drugs.** Depression pills reduce sexual drive and desire in the long term.
7. **Hip baths with anesthetic medicine or vaseline.** I know women who have burned their genitals because they could not adjust the heat while performing this homework, as well as women who pour these medicines

into the toilet bowl with hot water and who sit over them, getting serious genital infections…

8. **Botox application to the vagina.** As the problem occurs in the subconscious and as the lower vagina muscles are loose in Turkish women, this has no use.

9. **Single-session solution offers.** Learning is a process.

10. **Sexual intercourse trials in private clinics.** Having intercourse with other people present may cause trauma for the patient.

11. **Laceration at the muscle structure of the vagina.** It is not a solution since the problem is not with the vagina.

12. **EMDR on its own**: EMDR is a technique on traumas but it is deficient on its own.

13. **EFT**: EFT is a modified version of acupuncture, which has no place in vaginismus treatment.

14. **In Vitro Fertilization Clinics.** Treatments directed toward pregnancy cause the problem to be postponed without solution.

15. **Applying to religious functionaries with belief of being under a spell.** This is often seen in our society. Here is an anecdote on the matter. A patient is taken to a hodja. He listens and says, "Don't worry my girl; my daughter-in-law has the same problem. It has been one year and I'm about to solve it." ☺ This lights up ideas in our patient's mind and she runs out.

16. **Using aphrodisiac medicine.** Since vaginismus originates from fears and contractions, aphrodisiacs have no effect.

17. **NLP.** NLP is the simplified version of hypnosis. Its efficiency is less. R. Bandler, the founder of NLP, has tried to model M. Erickson's successful hypnosis sessions after his death by using language patterns. But even while he was alive, when asked about the secret to his success, M. Erickson had said, "Let me tell you with a story." As seen in his statement, the secret behind M. Erickson's success are *stories, anecdotes and metaphors.*

Due to the reasons provided, the above items don't have much place in vaginismus treatment. There could be a small patient group that has been healed with these methods. But it is my observation that the number of unhealed patients is much higher.

THINGS TO CONSIDER IN VAGINISMUS TREATMENT

The goal is to have intercourse. This is a simple phrase but the path to this simple sentence is a bit complicated. But why? Vaginismus is a mental, physical and emotional illness. To see vaginismus as only physical, or just mental or solely emotional, and to shape the treatment accordingly will be deficient. The most common mistake in treatments results from reducing this triple structure to single or double.

Approximately four out of ten hymens are elastic and non-bleeding membranes that allow penetration. Rarely, there are those that can cause problems and that need to be operated on. The remaining majority consist of membranes that also allow penetration but can have partial bleeding.

Physically, the hymen is not the only problem. Within the *Blue-Eyed Girl Effect* (Dr. Ulusoy definition. See Chapter Two, Dr. Ulusoy's Contributions to Vaginismus) some women -more common in Turkey- may have trouble tolerating something touching, pressuring or going inside. The reasons lying beneath this process are the helpless, unconfident and addictive structures in the personality, rather than physical structures.

At the same time, the habit of not urinating outside of home is commonly seen in women in Turkey, and sometimes OCD accompanies the situation. We have women who hold their urine for eight, twelve or even twenty-four hours. Interestingly, the vaginismus patients who have the habit of holding their urine for long periods also display serious problems of tolerating something going inside and increasing the diameter. Since the urinary bag cannot find any place to go in the front, it leans more onto the front vaginal wall at the rear. And because the urinary bag is rich with neural plexus and is also sensitive to tension, they have serious displeasure in case something penetrates into the vagina and increases its diameter. This displeasure can even lead all the way to fainting (Syncope). The reason for the fainting is the vaginal stimulation due to the pressures both from inside the vagina and also from the urinary bag. (Vaginal stimulation is the dizziness and fainting with the stimulation of parasympathetic system, thus causing bradycardia -reduction of heart rate- and reduction of its power to pump blood.)

When we examine the matter within the context of the mental and emotional structure, we see that, while learning information, the emotional contents of the information release dopamine (A kind of chemical inside the brain, also known as happiness hormone. Lack of it causes Parkinson's) at the amygdala in the brain, like pasting post-its, and they place the information inside the memory by marking information with emotions. The information that is marked with emotions is more easily remembered, and if this information + emotion chain includes fear, withdrawal or defense factors, such information is recalled in similar situations and the mind causes reactions in the body accordingly. In vaginismus, the cognitive distortions, dynamic structures or behaviorally experienced events coded with emotions in the past will involuntarily trigger bodily reactions.

A good vaginismus treatment should consist of methods that include all three structures. And a good formulation is required for the detection of the reasons of the problem. Formulations are different for each patient, and the treatment approaches will also differ according to these formulations. Lastly, the physician's experiences will become prominent in case of extra problems that may surface during treatment.

WHAT TO DO IN VAGINISMUS TREATMENT

We said that vaginismus is a *physical, mental and emotional* illness. In fact, this phrase defines the problem perfectly. Now that we have defined the problem clearly, the treatment needs to tackle this triple structure.

Some vaginismus women don't want to continue the treatment of the physical structure because of their fear of genital examination and because they are not in good terms with their genital region. The success rate in treatments done by neglecting the physical structure is relatively lower.

It is essential for the mental structure, the mind, to be educated at a certain level and in a way that the patient can understand, on the genital structure, the contents of the work (Mayalama), intercourse and positions.

And the emotional side of the matter includes the correction of the contractions, fear and panic symptoms, all which are the main reasons of vaginismus. At this point, a correct hypnosis technique will be useful. The physician needs to change the structure, which has been built toward withdrawal in the past, toward acceptance.

Moreover, the hypnosis method also helps the patient to come to terms with her genital area, to do her homework easily and to be able to have medical examinations easily.

As seen, the physician needs to provide the patient with the complete triple structure.

The man always needs to be included in the treatment process and he also needs to be informed during the education processes. The man should not display behavior or use words during the treatment that will upset his wife, or cause emotional refractions that will lead her to hopelessness. He should make an effort to keep his wife's motivation high.

Anecdote: Together with our patient, we completed our work for the day perfectly. I told them to rest for a night and that I would see them in the morning to carry out the therapy that would lead them to intercourse and that I would send them to the hotel for the experience. When our patient came in the next morning, she was pulling a long face. The couple was cross with each other. "What's up?" I asked, "Everything was fine yesterday, what happened?"

Our patient said, "Yesterday my husband told me that he didn't feel anything for me anymore. He said he felt things for other women but not for me!" Our entire treatment had gone to waste with these words of the husband. I asked them to repeat their homework once again; I somehow felt that the woman had not done it successfully yesterday.

Here, the existentialist structure in the woman had taken command, creating a reaction against the words of her husband. We arbitrated between them and overcame the problem during the day. In any case, I tell my patients this, "Our treatment hours are very precious. Never show negative behavior to each other. Let me complete your treatment successfully, you have your intercourse, and you are free to throw dishes and vases at each other when you go home later." ☺

Since the treatment process is mainly intended toward the woman and it is directed toward education, the vaginismus woman should do her best to understand, perceive and apply the physician's advice and practices.

When difficulties are met during treatment, she should not say, "I want to stop treatment, I cannot continue." The vaginismus woman should realize that this is her problem. If she leaves the treatment halfway, she will have failed and she will be burdened with the responsibility of the problems she will have with her husband in the future.

A sympathetic husband during vaginismus is one who leads his wife to treatment without wasting any time. At the same time, if his wife ever wants to stop the treatment and tells him that she wants to go, he should be able to say,

"We are here to get cured and you should do your best to try and do whatever the doctor suggests."

An understanding man is not the one that says, "Let's leave it to time," or who says, "Okay honey, you just don't worry. Let's stop the treatment and go home," when his wife wants to quit.

It should not be forgotten that we are working on the woman's fears, helplessness and weak self during vaginismus treatment, and if the man does not provide enough support during this process, the treatment will fail or remain deficient.

Vaginismus treatment includes working on the vagina, building friendship with the genital area, and removing fear, panic and contractions. Within the entire content of the treatment, actually, the vaginismus patient is being offered a model regarding intercourse. It is this model that we expect the vaginismus patient to learn, understand and apply.

When the vaginismus woman is directed toward intercourse, she step-by-step carries out the experience by following and applying the model that we have taught her.

From this point of view, every patient that comes in for vaginismus treatment needs to have sufficient competence in *learning, understanding and application*.

The process contains a model similar to that of learning how to drive.

As I have presented during the congress, it is possible to complete this entire process in a short period of time (A day and a half on average).

We frequently receive this question from our patients, "What kind of differences are there with longer lasting treatments?" or "What is it that you do so the patient can reach the solution so quickly?"

The most accurate and basic answer to both questions is that we are aware of the necessity of realizing that vaginismus is a physical, mental and emotional illness, and that we plan the treatment accordingly. Most probably, this structure is not completely conformed to in long-term treatments so the process is prolonged due to incomplete structures during the treatment.

Another important point is that vaginismus treatment should not be seen solely as behavioral; meaning that instead of trying to reach the solution by directly working on the vagina, one should plan the treatment with *cognitive, behavioral and hypnotherapy* processes in conformity with the triple structure I have mentioned above, while knowing that every woman's vaginismus problem will vary according to her personality structure and ethiology, and by structuring the treatment with the best formulation suitable for her.

A separate formulation must be done for each patient according to,
1. Cognitive reasons,
2. Behavioral reasons,
3. Dynamic reasons,
4. Existentialist reasons.

Then, it would be best to organize the treatment according to the reasons specific to the patient. Afterwards, based on the identified problems, hypnotherapy will be practiced by focusing on *problem* + emotion.

ADDITIONAL INFORMATION IN VAGINISMUS TREATMENT

1. If a vaginismus patient has thalassemia major (Mediterranean anemia where she receives blood each month) or any other diseases with bleeding defect, we suggest that you operate on her hymen in a hospital before taking your patient into therapy. Otherwise, you may face serious problems during her solo finger exercises and works with devices, or during the intercourse trial in case the hymen is deformed and bleeds.
2. If your vaginismus patient has suffered a serious sexual trauma in the past, you need to be alert for disassociations and split personalities during therapy.
3. If there are conversions together with vaginismus, one needs to pay attention to conversive episodes during therapy.
4. If your vaginismus patient has continence problems affiliated to OCD, it is important to be cautious about the neurogenic bladder during penetration into the vagina with anything.
5. As the vagina tissue is open to vagal stimulation, one should keep an eye open during penetration into vagina by anything (Finger, device, penis) for bradycardia and syncope related to vagal stimulation.
6. If there is a septate (Two partitions, double ringed) hymen or if the hymen is sieve type or with a small and narrow entrance, the hymen needs to be operated.
7. If your vaginismus patient or her partner has schizoid, schizophrenic or paranoid mental disorders, the therapy needs to be carried out carefully and cautiously.

8. Your vaginismus patient and her partner need to know in advance that the hymen could become deformed during the exercises they will perform, and that they may not have the chance to leave the hymen deformation until the first experience.

9. Similarly, they also need to know that four out of ten hymens are elastic and allow penetration, and that it may not bleed during exercises or intercourse trials.

10. The therapist has to know that vaginas may vary in length, inclination and diameter.

11. The Bartholin Cyst is a reason that causes pain during sexual intercourse, and it may be mistaken as vaginismus by the patient.

12. As penis curvature also makes vaginal penetration difficult, it could also be interpreted by the patient or her partner as vaginismus.

13. If the vaginismus woman is married and her husband is not keen on treatment, and if the woman applies to you with her lover for treatment, it will be appropriate for you to decline. Otherwise, you may face legal problems.

14. It is important to keep video recordings and files of vaginismus patients, and to safely store your work and your archives. You may be asked legally for information years later in case of future problems between spouses.

15. Vaginismus patients always seek certainty, clarity and guarantee. Do not abuse such expectations of the patients for monetary gain. Unfortunately, there are many patients who have applied to many such places and who have been left halfway. Such patients become disheartened and are unable to trust anyone. First of all, remember the principle "Do not harm…" But ethically, no matter how good and successful you are in the treatment, share with your patient the risks, possibilities and the actions to be taken. And before starting the treatment, have these signed by the patient on an *informed consent form* (Chapter 2, Sample informed consent form).

16. If, by chance, a patient becomes impregnated during the trials and if she wants to have vaginismus treatment during her pregnancy, we need to accept them into treatment at least six months after the birth in order to prevent the risk of miscarriage, puerperal infections and depression.

DO KEGEL EXERCISES HAVE A PLACE IN VAGINISMUS TREATMENT?

Kegel Exercises are frequently used in Turkey and abroad for vaginismus treatment. It is assumed that that the lower 1/3 of vaginal muscles are contracting and exercising of the lower pelvic floor (Pubococcygeus – PC) muscles for that region are prescribed. With this exercise, it is aimed to provide control in the pelvic floor muscles and to allow penis penetration. The patient is asked to do these exercises in a sitting position and as long as she can do them throughout the day, or to perform a set number of repetitions three or four times a day.

In brief summary, this exercise comprises of the application of the holding and releasing action done while urinating, without actually urinating. Some women mistakenly do this while urinating.

In fact, this exercise has three areas where it is effective.
1. In the vaginismus cases seen in foreign countries, which do not originate from first night fright but which are developed afterwards because of pelvic floor muscles.
2. In women who develop enuresis problems after a certain age and who develop urinary incontinence.
3. It can also be used after the penis-vagina trials have been competed to enable the woman to learn how to use these muscles and give more pleasure to her partner and to herself.

My own studies, observations and experiences have shown that Kegel Exercises have no place in the vaginismus seen in Turkey. Unfortunately, they are still widely used because of the therapists' lack of knowledge and experience.

These homeworks sometimes cause the patient to move away from treatment because this is what she thinks, "I completely do the homework my doctor gives me, I even did extra Kegel Exercises in my seat but I still can't have intercourse."

Therefore, it is much more efficient in the treatment to see from where the problem originates and to work directly toward the problem. Kegel Exercises may be suggested after the treatment to increase the comfort and pleasure of intercourse, there is no harm in this.

VAGINISMUS ETIOLOGY AND THE ROLE OF THE PSOAS MUSCLES IN TREATMENT

The Psoas Muscle is the keystone of a balanced body. It is a large muscle at about 17-20 inches in length. It connects the thorax and torso to the legs. There is one at each side of the torso, comprised of Psoas Major and Psoas Minor. It originates from the T12 vertebra and continues as it exits from the L1 to L5 vertebrae. The Psoas Major passes through the pelvis, over the hip socket and connects to the splint at the inner edge of the femur (Lesser trochanter). The Psoas does not connect directly to the pelvis. It plays vital role on the pelvis with its relation with the thorax and the femur, more importantly with the tendon that it connects to with the Iliacus muscle over the femur. The Psoas and Iliacus are jointly known as Iliopsoas. The location of the Psoas effects the relationships between the organs, diaphragm, the blood circulation system and the nervous system. The Psoas has fascia connections with the diaphragm at the top, and with the pelvic floor muscles at the bottom. This way, it controls the pressure at the lumbar region and supports the balance and strength of this region. The tonus and quality of the Psoas Muscle effects the pelvis and all the organs inside that area. In a team effort with the diaphragm and the abdominal muscles, the contraction and relaxation of the Psoas massages the inner organs, stimulates blood circulation and influences the general health of the organs.

The diaphragm is a muscle structure that separates the chest from the abdomen. The liver, stomach and spleen inside the abdominal cavity are on its lower surface, while the heart is right on top of it. It is the primary muscle of respiration. Just as the Psoas, the diaphragm is effected by both the skeleton and also the by rhythms of the inner organ structures, and it responds to these rhythms. As it moves up and down, it not only massages the organs but also massages the vertebrae and provides the synovial fluid's flow from the spinal column to the brain.

The pelvic floor muscles are a hammock-shaped muscle group between the pubis, the sitting muscles and the tip of the sacrum that carry the torso from its lower end. With the angle it creates while passing over the hip joint, the Psoas acts as a shelf and helps the pelvic floor in carrying the lower abdominal organs and also in carrying the baby during pregnancy.

The lumbar neural network is a complex nerve net that passes through and around the Psoas. Many nerves are buried inside the Psoas surface. The complex communication between the organs in the abdominal region and the brain also includes the Psoas. By twisting certain vertebrae, the Psoas replies or interprets messages. The nerves at the lumbar region may be thought of as our abdominal brain. The Psoas is located in the area of the abdominal region where instinctive emotions are felt. The upper tip of the Psoas and the diaphragm join at the solar plexus.

The Psoas follows a parallel path along the lowering aorta and the lumbar and hip regions. It influences the blood flow to the lower body and it is affected by it. The kidneys are at the side of the Psoas, while the bladder and reproductive organs lie in front of it. The fascia tissue of the kidneys and the fascia tissue of the Psoas are so intertwined that they seem to be one and unitary. During an operation on either of them, it is inevitable for the connective tissue of the other one to be affected.

Functions of the Psoas Muscle

Psoas, generally depicted as hip flexor, is much more than that. The main function of the Psoas is to provide free oscillation of the leg while walking, and it plays a role in transferring the load from the body to the legs and feet. Walking and running are not actions that originate at the legs, but on the contrary, that originate from the center of the torso. The Psoas responds to the gravitational changes in the torso and the legs follow it (Koch, 2012).

The Psoas acts as a guide wire that stabilizes the spine (Just like the side wires that support the main pole of a tent). At the same time, the Psoas serves as a support for the organs; its liveliness, health and length trigger the organs' functions. The organs having an area inside the pelvis, where they can rest comfortably and function normally, depends on the length and tonus of the Psoas Muscle.

The Psoas and erector spinae muscles are in correlation. The erector spinae muscles are located behind the spine and they are mostly weak. But while the Psoas is in resting position and at natural resting length, the erector spinae muscles reach the tonus that can support the load of the ribcage. Strengthening these muscles will free the Psoas.

Psoas plays a balancing role for the rectus abdominis muscles (front-rear relationship). The balance between these two muscles provides a feeling of wholeness. Sit-ups and similar exercises not only slim the Psoas but also tightens and shortens it, thus loading extra stress on the waist muscles that are mostly under extreme load, and also on the diaphragm and the internal organs. The natural harmony and rhythm is lost and the person sees himself only as his body.

Finally, Psoas serves as a hydraulic pump. Such movement triggers the flow of fluids in and out of the cells. The Psoas Muscle, which contracts and stretches during normal walk, is active and its normal movement constantly stimulates the organs and the spine. Due to the fact that it is a free moving muscle rather than a structural support, Psoas assists constant and unhindered blood flow from the main arteries to the legs and feet. The Psoas and lumbar neural network directly provide the energy that mobilizes the legs, and it also has important role in activating anal and sexual functions.

The psychological functions of the Psoas Muscles are recently being recognized in the field. Whereas in reality, this is one of the oldest knowledge of human history. Yoga, in particular, shows us that the ancient wise men had perceived the importance of the Psoas Muscle centuries ago. Many of the yoga poses practiced around the World today are based on the principle of extending and stretching of the Psoas Muscle. And this provides physical and mental relaxation, and reduces anxiety.

Psoas and Fear Reflex

Apart from the thighbone, the Psoas Muscle also connects to the diaphragm. The diaphragm muscle, which moves during breathing, is also an area where many physical symptoms related to fear and anxiety take place. Liz Koch thinks that this is directly related with the Psoas and also with the brain stem and the "reptilian brain" which is the oldest known part of the spinal cord. According to Koch, long before the spoken word or the organizing capacity of the cortex developed, the reptilian brain, known for its survival instincts, maintained our essential core functioning (Koch, 2012).

The only fear that is instinctive and not related to personal experience is the fear of falling. It occurs with a complex set of neural messages and results in the contraction of the flexor muscles. As one of the largest flexor muscles, Psoas is activated immediately with fear. The fear reflex is formed early in the first week of life and settles into our nerve-muscle system. When we hear a very loud sound or when we are caught unpreparedly by a situation that is likely to give us physical pain, the body assumes a state of protection. The head is drawn down between the shoulders, the shoulders rise toward the ears, the abdominal and hip flexor muscles contract, and the muscles at the back of the body stiffen.

The Psoas Muscle contracts whenever the fear reflex is triggered. By doing so, its tips come closer to each other, creating a closure that gives the feeling of safety, and thus covers and secures the soft, vulnerable areas (Genital organs, vital organs, and the face). Fight or flight is a stimulation that effects the entire body; the sympathetic nervous system kicks into action and the heartbeat and breathing speed up with the secretion of adrenaline. Under normal circumstances, when the threat is removed, the parasympathetic nervous system returns to its original state with the relaxation of all these muscles.

When the fear reflex is constantly repeated without balancing resting periods and solution (flight or fight), or if it constantly repeats in short bursts, a conditioned reaction that creates constant tension in order to keep the body ready for the next fear reflex/attack. This is experienced as tension anxiety.

The main problems in vaginismus are fear and contraction, closure and withdrawal related to intercourse. No matter if classical information describes contraction at the lower 1/3 of vaginal muscles -pubococcygeal pelvic floor muscles- it is not always the case. Kegel Exercises are directed at training the lower vagina (Pelvic floor) muscles. Whereas the vagina, the pelvic floor muscles, are loose in vaginismus. The main problem in vaginismus is the contraction -with fear and by means of the diaphragm/breathing- of the Psoas Muscles that are under the control of the primitive area of the brain.

The main reasons why the treatment duration has been reduced down to three hours in The Dr. Ulusoy Method are the following.
- The elimination of fear with hypnosis
- Enabling control of the Psoas Muscles with hypnosis and feedback-supported exercises
- Providing bodily relaxation with hypnosis
- Speeding of learning with hypnosis

By enabling diaphragm control with the breathing technique that includes holotropic and leg feedback-assisted mindfulness during examination and exercise, the protective, evasive primitive reflex at the brain stem related to intercourse is controlled, and also the relaxation of the Psoas Muscles, and consequently of the femurs, is provided.

REASONS OF FAILURE IN VAGINISMUS TREATMENT

Although there are many reasons for the failures in vaginismus treatment, it is possible to list the main topics as follows.

A. Reasons concerning the physician

1. Vaginismus treatment may require vaginal exercises. If the treatment is carried out not by physicians but by therapists or psychiatrists that to not perform examination or exercise, it may remain incomplete. Because psychologists and psychiatrists apply classical treatment. Classical treatments rely heavily on homework and when the patient does not do her homework, the treatment becomes unsustainable. Or the patient may do the homework but the trial does not happen anyway.
2. The lack of the physician's knowledge, practice and experience regarding vaginismus treatment.
3. Attempting to deal with a high number of patients at the same time could also lead to failure.

B. Reasons concerning the patient

1. The patient's unwillingness.
2. The patient not loving her partner.
3. The patient thinking of divorce.
4. The patient being in love with another man.
5. The patient rejecting to be treated.
6. Incapability of the patient to learn and understand.

C. Reasons concerning the patient's partner

1. The partner preventing the woman from being examined.
2. The partner's desire for the hymen to be deformed during the first intercourse and his rejection of the treatment.
3. The partner using psychological or physical violence against the woman in the past and/or during the treatment period.

D. Reasons due to the efficiency of the therapy method or due to the practical competence of the therapy method, or of the therapist against problems that may occur during treatment

Milton Erickson was a therapist who trusted and believed in himself to the point that he had said, "If you can't do it, I can." And most of the time, he would take active role in order to reach his patient's mind and to change it. But in most of the therapies of our time, and especially in the classical vaginismus treatments, the therapist usually leaves the patient alone with regards to homework and exercises to be done. When the patient says, "I couldn't do it," the process is prolonged or the treatment is resulted in failure.

QUESTIONS AND ANSWERS

Q: How successful is the next sexual intercourse after the first intercourse takes place under hypnosis? I ask because I think vaginismus is a psychological illness and it is only the first intercourse that takes place under hypnosis...

A: As you think, vaginismus is a psychological product of defective learning. After solving the problem in the subconscious, you experience the first intercourse. This first experience does not take place under hypnosis, as I understand you suggest in your question. Only your misinformation (Knowingly or not) is corrected with hypnotic suggestions while hypnotized. So, when you have the first experience, your conscious is open and you are aware of everything. After that? Just as you don't require driving training every time you want to drive after learning how to drive a car, the future sexual experiences occur easily, since your subconscious has been programmed with new teachings.

Q: Vaginismus was a serious problem I experienced when I first got married. I was unable to be with my husband for ten months. We had come to the point of divorce so I decided to see a physician about it. He gave me two pills, a numbing spray and a cream for me to use before having sex. We were able to have intercourse with the help of these things. But unfortunately, I have been married for two and a half years, and I still suffer unbearable pain each time. As I still clamp myself, I am devastated by the pain when my husband's penis enters me. He tried to inch it in slowly and of course he loses concentration and I feel nothing but pain. I am always scared that my husband will come and want to have sex, and this makes him very unhappy. What I want to know is whether this hypnosis will make it possible for me not to feel pain, or for me not to see this as torture but as something enjoyable like other people feel. Could you help me with this? Thanks in advance for your time.

A. As we always say, vaginismus originates from the subconscious. Drugs and sedation may provide intercourse for that one time. As for the problem of the subconscious, we can solve it with hypnosis, which is an altered state of consciousness. Since sexuality is an instinctive nature of mankind, with hypnosis we not only enable intercourse, but also make it possible for you to experience intercourses that reach unproblematic satisfaction by feeling sexual desire and pleasure. At the same time, after the therapy, you will also have learned how to use your mind and your subconscious, meaning that you can control yourself, your contractions.

Q: I have been married for five years, I've been together with my husband for six years but I still haven't had intercourse with him… From the articles I've read online, I was thinking that I had vaginismus, but I was able to have a voluntary sexual relationship in the third year of my marriage with someone else and it lasted for a year. But my lack of sexual appetite for my husband still continues. Do you think my problem could be solved with hypnosis treatment?

A: As also evident in your story, the subconscious factor is once again beneath the vaginismus problem. You cannot have intercourse with your husband but you are able to have sex with someone else. Knowingly or unknowingly (Subthreshold learning), you have developed an aversion toward your husband. It is of course possible to reach a solution with hypnotherapy if you wish to do so. The solution will come by investigating the problem and by supporting you with positive suggestions.

Q: I am a virgin and I have not had any attempts to change this situation, but I think I had experienced vaginismus in my previous trials. I don't want to let someone into my life before solving this problem, but I also don't know how I can solve this problem without being with a man. I desperately need an advice that I can accept.

A: You have probably had fears and contractions in your previous experiences. We can provide education to remove your fear and contractions. After this education, you will be feeling much more comfortable. Most probably your problem will be solved. But in case you have any problems during a future coupling, we can solve the problem completely with a short therapy at that time.

Q: I've surfed your website quite a lot and I read the positive comments of your previous patients on hypnotherapy. But I noticed that the women who have posted comments are those who have had sexual problems since their first sexual experiences. I wonder if this therapy is applicable for my case. I am thirty-five years old. I didn't have any sexual problems until three years ago. But a short while ago, I learned from my gynecologist that I was suffering from minor vaginismus. We are quite happy with my husband. We don't fight, nor do we have a boring life. Why did this come from out of the blue? Do you think hypnotherapy could be applied for my case too?

A: It's an interesting situation. The result of the examination is not what counts. It is the quality of your relationship with your husband. If you still don't have problems in the intercourse due to the penis-vagina relationship, you don't need therapy. If you have slight problems, we can find a solution with hypnotherapy. Besides, hypnotherapy could boost the pleasure you take from sex...

Q: About one and a half years ago, I was subjected to severe harassment. Now, I have a relationship that is getting better each day but I am unable to be with my husband because of the experienced I suffered. I have fears that I have not overcome. I stat trembling even when I hear something about sex, I get nauseous, my muscles contract. I want to get rid of this. I would really appreciate it if you could help me. Good day...

A: I understand your problem. With hypnotherapy, it is possible to solve this distress that has settled into your subconscious. At the same time, it is also possible to enable you to take pleasure from intercourse and to have a quality climax, rather than just having a mechanical relationship.

Q: Hello Mr. Murat. There was some pain in my left groin for five months and as you would imagine, I could not go to a physician. I called an expert gynecologist here and explained her the situation. She told me to take an appointment and come over. I prepared myself and went there. First she talked for a while and said that it would heal with treatment. Then she looked at my abdomen on the ultrasound machine and said that I had a cyst in my right ovary. Then she asked if we should take a look at my hymen. She made me so relaxed and she behaved so nice that I said, "Yes." I lied down in that chair and she looked at my hymen. She told me that the right side of my hymen was completely torn and that the left side was partially torn. She comforted me and said that she wanted to palpate me there and that she wouldn't do it if I didn't want to. She said she just wanted to look. And I thought I had to start from somewhere and accepted it. She prepped me without showing the ultrasound device and looked inside. Of course I convulsed a bit but she was so reassuring that I managed it. Then we sat and started talking. I was so happy for being able to get examined. That had been almost impossible for me. But while talking, I suddenly began to glaze over and got nauseous. I said nothing, thinking that it would pass. But then I fainted at the spot. I woke up with my legs up high and my head being cologned on the wall. My tension during the examination resulted in my blood pressure dropping. The physician lady said that there was a psychiatrist at the upper floor, that the four other patients she had sent there had been healed and that they had given normal births. She said she would call and tell him about my situation if I said okay. Besides, she told me that I didn't have any physiological problems and that my problem was totally psychological. After resting for a while, I went upstairs and met with the doctor. I said I wanted to be rid of this and began treatment. Actually I was not keen on being treated here but that was how events occurred. The doctor told me that, if I didn't respond to this treatment, he would send me to a friend of his for hypnosis treatment. I hope I will succeed in the treatment and be rid of this. I wanted to tell you about these beforehand. In fact, I wanted to come to you but I thought I should try this doctor first. I await your comments. Hope to see you again, good day...

A: Although you have allowed physical examination, later you have experienced a manifestation of an inner tension originating from fear. Normally, in order to overcome your problem, it is advised that you take a therapy which is effective on mental processes directed toward the subconscious. But it is also advised that ongoing treatments should not be quitted in any case. Please continue seeing the psychiatrist you have gone to. If you are unable to have results, ask the hypnotherapist you will be sent to about the techniques he will apply to you. As I have frequently written in the past, the hypnotherapist and the techniques he applies are very important. Hypnosis on its own is like a syringe; the important thing is the medicine that will be put into the syringe to cure you. If you receive only relaxation, loosening and fear removal suggestions, the therapy may be deficient. Please read once again the previous messages on our Yahoo Group and also the information on our web site, and if necessary, find out what methods the hypnotherapist you plan to see will be using. I hope that your problem will be solved quickly by your psychiatrist and that you enjoy sexuality...

Q: I am currently unable to have intercourse. I have been married for three and a half years, and we could say that we had intercourse -not fully- two times with long periods between them. It has been almost a year since the last time. There are still no improvements since that one year. We can't have intercourse. If my problem is vaginismus; could I still be able to have those two experiences? That is what I wanted to ask. Thank you. Best regards...

A: Your problem can be evaluated as vaginismus. But it is a fluctuating vaginismus; although you can have sex from time to time, you can't have a natural sexuality. It is probably originating from fears and anxieties, or there is another mechanism in your subconscious. Hypnotherapy is advised in such case. Your problem is vaginismus. The fact that it allows intercourse in long intervals does not prove that it is not vaginismus...

Q: Hello doctor! I am married for six years and I have an eight-month-old son. It hurts when I have sex with my husband. It is more like torture than pleasure. I am not comfortable; I strain myself during intercourse. Am I some kind of vaginismus patient? Could hypnosis be a cure?

A: You are able have vaginal intercourse. This shows that you don't have vaginismus. But the fact that you strain yourself and feel distress instead of pleasure could be corrected with hypnotherapeutic visualization and you will feel pleasure and reach satisfaction during sex. Probably, your problem originates from sex-related fears and anxieties nestled in your subconscious. Your situation can also be seen in vaginismus cases that have been insufficiently treated without the contractions being removed completely.

Q: I am twenty-six year-old woman, married for eleven months. We have been together with my husband for six years but we have not been able to have sex although we tried many times. First we thought it was vaginismus because there were contractions and severe pain during all our trials. In a regular physician examination, we found out that my hymen was elastic, thick and fleshy. I was told that my hymen needed to be torn with an operation. Unfortunately we have not been able to have the operation yet due to the medical facilities at the place we are right now. There were no contractions in our latest trials; I am quite comfortable but the only problem is the pain! I am not afraid to have sex, I am not someone raised with sexual taboos. But when I read your web site, I started having question marks in my mind again. I have a question for you: Do you think my problem could be vaginismus? Or is it my hymen? Thanks in advance. ☺

A: Usually, the first thing that gynecologists say about vaginismus is that there are problems with the hymen and their first advice is an operation. Whereas hymens that don't allow penetration are quite rare as literature suggests. They think that everything will be easy once the hymen is removed. And this is a result of a two-dimensional approach to the three-dimensional human being. The important thing is not the removal of the mechanical obstacle in front of the problem, but the necessity to solve the mental obstacle. Unfortunately, most of the cases we receive come with an operation of the hymen but they are unable to have sex. The fact that you had contractions and pain in your previous trials, but that the contractions have disappeared recently is a good sign. You write that you feel pain nonetheless. If the contraction does not originate from the lower vagina muscles, the hymen operation could be suitable for you. If there is still pain and ache after the hymen operation, then the problem could be removed with sessions. The terms elastic, thick and fleshy are a bit vague. If it is elastic, penetration is easy. The hymen that does not allow penetration has to be stiff and needs to have the structure and size that prevents penis penetration.

Q: Hello Mr. Murat. I found your address in the *Sizinle* magazine. I am three-months married and vaginismus is my problem too. ☺ I feel grateful as I read the cases here because I am at the early times of my marriage and there are people who suffer from this for seven-eight years! I said I was married for three months but we are together with my husband since four years and we experienced everything other than a complete sexual intercourse. I mean we made love but I was always nervous because I felt I was betraying my beliefs. Our first trial was on our wedding night and I could not do it. I felt a lot of pain. And we tried the second one on our honeymoon, thinking that we were very tired then so we should try it now. Again, it didn't happen. My husband is really very understanding. I am currently in search of treatment. I want to ask a few things about this. From what you say, this is a psychological thing. So, would it be a solution to see a psychologist? Or is hypnosis preferred because it is a quicker solution? And, how will you determine if I am suitable for hypnosis or not?

A: Hello. As you have also seen on our web site and in our group, there are plenty of methods. It is up to you to choose the method. I advise you to pick whichever method sounds plausible to you, whichever you trust. Because trust is an important factor in treatment. Vaginismus is psychological but my answer about it being solved with a psychiatrist would be as follows. The foundation is very important, almost everyone in Turkey says they can handle it and therapies are continued for months. And when you stop and look back, you see that you have not achieved anything at all, as you can see in the mails sent to the group... Over the years, our patients go to this psychiatrist or that psychologist and they are whisked around. We find solutions with our hypnotherapeutic approach. Hypnotherapy is not preferred only for its quickness but also for its assistance in terms of your pleasure and perception. As the method is directly focused on the subconscious, the solution comes quickly. Treatment is a matter of correct education and process. In the end, you will not remain this way and you will be able to experience sex with the best sense of pleasure...

Q: Hello, I am married for two years and unfortunately I am also a vaginismus patient. I am a member of the group and I am scared even to send a message. There is not such a therapy center in the city we live in. I was treated in another city one year ago but I got no results, we were left at the penis penetration stage. You are very much involved with the people in the group, something that I was not unable to get from the other physician. I called him to say that penis penetration did not happen. He said, "It will, try again." And I could not call afterwards, and he never called me back either. One year has passed since. Everything is the same. My husband keeps saying we will do it but we can't even try. I can't tell my husband that I want to come and see you because the travel expenses and the treatment costs at the other place were so high. I know he will say, "No, we'll manage it." But he isn't aware of the passing time. I don't know what to do. At the place I went before, they first made a vagina examination, like straining and loosening the muscles. Then he kept talking to me psychologically. Then I had a treatment in which I inserted first my pinky, then my ring finger and finally my husband's finger into my vagina. As I said, I stopped at the penis penetration phase; only the head was able to enter, we could not do the rest. Please help me; what am I do to? I have nobody to support me. My husband says we'll do it, but time is passing by. I want to be a mother already. Help me...

A: Believe me; there is so little left for you to succeed. Your husband is partially right. You have actually benefitted from the physician you've been to. You are able to perform finger controls. And when your fear of intercourse is solved with the hypnotherapeutic method that we will apply, you will have no more problems and you will be a great mother... We call our therapy patients at every stage for support and we try to reply, as best as we can, all the questions of the members of our group. We know that your problem will be solved easily with a good therapy and with support that does not allow you to feel left alone.

Q: Hi there. I am married for fourteen months and I have vaginismus. Apparently it is not an illness but I am losing hope because my husband doesn't agree to see a physician. It is really difficult to remain married this way. I await your help on this matter. And also, what are the chances that you can cure this in one session with hypnosis?

A: Please let all our men read this message.

Your wife's situation is psychological. Please don't despise her for her illness; be by her side, support her but let this support be more than pity. Your support should not be saying, "Okay honey, let's not do it," when she hurts a little. Every moment that you don't do it, that you don't try it, will solidify the negativity. It may not be that day but you can try it some other time. Create different environments that will force changes in the conscious, make her feel the romance, cherish her feelings. And don't try sudden trials to make everything go away immediately. Help her relax with your touches, words and kisses. Her whole body will relax with the right approach. Let her feel safe in your arms, let her desire sex. Imagine you are directing a movie and imagine that you are together with a fairy in this movie. Assume that your wife is a princess in a frog's body; she will become the most beautiful woman with your kisses, and the vaginismus problem will go away…

Both the man and the woman should first try to recognize, to feel each other's genital structures by touching. Finally, this is a therapy, not something that can be built in a day. We are able to cure vaginismus in three phases and approximately one and a half days.

Q: Hello. It has been nine months since we got married. I am having vaginismus problem. I have done quite a lot of research on the matter. I guess psychological treatment is necessary for it to be healed. My husband is very understanding about this matter. He always tries to help me. He offered to see a physician and found you during his research. The first thing I want to know is; if this is an 80% psychological problem, could I overcome it with my own efforts? Could I progress with the suggestions I give to myself. I don't know the method but I want to try to solve it by myself first. If it doesn't work, of course I will seek professional help. But like I said, what do you think are the odds for me to beat this on my own? I wish you success in your work; I read that you are really helping people. Thank you in advance…

A: If your problem is a simple vaginismus, if it is not based on the dynamics of the subconscious, I mean, if it is comprised only of simple fear and tension, you may try to overcome it with the method we call self-hypnosis. In fact, there are three types of hypnosis.

1. **Heterohypnosis** which is done with the mediation of a hypnotherapist.
2. **Autohypnosis** which is the situation created by the new conditioned reflexes given by the therapist.
3. **Self-hypnosis** which is the situation that is comprised of the suggestions the person gives to herself unknowingly throughout the day.

This is what I tell to vaginismus patients who characteristically always focus on the negatives. "*If you look out of the window and see a man who constantly trips himself and falls down, I guess you would laugh at him. But you are also tripping yourself constantly with negative thoughts and beliefs.*"

And sometimes, while we are giving education in the first phase of the treatment, the vaginismus patient is there bodily but her mind is not. She is as if in a bell glass. She sees us but cannot hear us. She is wandering in her inner reality that is formed by her own cognitive distortions. At that moment, I stop the training and ask, "*I think you're not here, am I right?*" Our patient is startled for a moment and realizes that the therapist is monitoring herself, her emotions and her inner chaos. With this approach, I am able to build a bond of trust between the patient and myself. "I am with you, I am by your side, I feel what you feel. *Trust me; I will get you out of this bottomless pit.*"

The things you can do on your own are the following.

1. Be courageous
2. Believe that you will succeed
3. Start by believing, wait with confidence
4. Touch your genital structures with your husband, both the penis and the vagina. Feel them…
5. Lie down on your back and take deep breaths. Do this at least twenty minutes a day. Strain and the relax yourself, starting from your toes and move toward your neck in succession.
6. Use the Kegel Exercises in further stages, to increase pleasure after the trial.
7. When you lie in your bed at night, close your eyes and dream of your intercourse with your husband. Respond to your dream with your body. Feel…

And finally, if you are unable to get any results from these exercises, apply for therapy. You will be coming prepared if you do these exercises. Let us solve the vicious circle that you are trapped in your subconscious with the methods we will apply…

Q: First of all, thank you for replying my question. You said, "If you have a simple vaginismus…" How can I understand if this is a simple one or not? Are there any ways to measure? Does my lack of sexual desire also originate from this illness? I don't need sex in any way, nor do I want it. How can I overcome this? Is this something that can also be done with suggestions? Or do I need medical treatment? And another thing; do the medicine that enhance sexual power and desire (Herbal-chemical) provide any help in vaginismus treatment? How healthy is it to use such things? Thanks again. Best regards…

A: If you have not experienced a sexual trauma in your past and if you are able to control the vagina entrance and the inside of the vagina, but if you have contractions during intercourse, if you tremble and push your husband away, this is a relatively easy situation to solve. Lack of sexual drive does not directly come from vaginismus but prolonging the period in which vaginismus is not cured could cause the development of deficient sexual desire due to abstinence. Also, unwillingness due to repugnance could also lead up to vaginismus. There could be many reasons for your lack of sexual desire.

1. A hormonal imbalance
2. Perception of sex as dirty, filthy or bad
3. Sexual trauma
4. Indifference toward the partner
5. Lack of instinct

If the problem is not hormonal, hypnotherapy takes first place among treatment options. The causes are investigated, sexual desire is aroused with suggestions and orgasm is introduced.

There are many substances and medicine in the market that increase sexual potency. I would not like to suggest any medicine for you but you can provide this with natural food. Deserts, cream, walnuts, honey, bananas, peanut butter, pistachio butter and chocolate are aphrodisiac food. By the way, please watch out for your weight. ☺ While such food will increase your sexual desires, they have no direct effect in solving vaginismus; they provide indirect assistance…

A plate with some honey in the middle and some cream on top of it, and on top of the cream, some crushed walnuts and pistachios, and some fleshy banana slices around it all could be a nice menu to have with a couple of glasses of wine… There's a great aphrodisiac for you! You will feel the warming inside; the widening of your veins and you will feel you are ready to share something with your partner… (Should I quit vaginismus treatments and become a gourmet?)

I thank you for making me feel another point of view… When I was setting up our vaginismus treatment site, I could never have thought that I would be able to provide support for people in such a wide range of topics. I will try to answer all of your questions to the best of my knowledge, as best as I can…

Q: Thank you for your support. Frankly speaking, I was not sure I would be getting such regular answers since my first e-mail. I also thank you for showing us that not everything is done for a benefit.

I did not feel the need to research anything about sex before I got married. I thought I could learn everything by experience. So much that I was not aware that I did not know my own body. I realized this after getting married. It's very funny but I never knew, nor did I even look where the vagina was, where the urethra was…

Perhaps this was why I could not have intercourse in the beginning. I was afraid I would do something wrong because I didn't know how. After realizing this, I began to examine myself. It was not so severe at first, I was clamping myself but perhaps it was not at a level that would prevent intercourse. Now I feel it has advanced; do you think this illness progresses if not treated? When I opened my e-mail inbox I came across a mail on the topic that was exactly what I was going to ask you. I had done a lot of online research about the hymen. I had also seen ones with pictures. And I used some means of technology to look at mine. One imagines something thin when thinking about the hymen but it was as if I was looking at a huge chunk of flesh. ☺ And I could not liken its shape to any that I had seen. It seemed to be completely closed and just had a small opening at the right side. So tiny that it was hardly seen. Perhaps it looked like the ones you call half-moon. But I would be lying if I said I wasn't afraid to see it. "If it is so thick and if the opening is so small, it will hurt me a lot," I said to myself. Maybe I never should have looked, right? Is it possible to understand by looking if the hymen is thick or whether it is at a level that it will hurt or not? Thank you…

A: As time goes by, negative beliefs may develop with each failed trial. It is nice that you know yourself. But don't overestimate that piece of flesh. Don't forget that a four-inch head of a baby can fit through that entrance you think to be too small. I mean, the hymen and the vagina have elastic structures. The hymen will not hurt, your fear will. Believe me…

Q: I have been married for three years and we haven't had intercourse yet. I am so frightened. I even tried to get drunk to have sex, but in vain. I am very scared that it will hurt. We don't have the financial means to see a psychologist. So I can't have treatment either. My husband has been very understanding until now but he has recently begun frowning and talking sarcastically. I don't have the right to be angry with him because he has waited long enough. After all, he's a man; he has the right to be mad. But I don't want to lose him. I don't feel like a woman anymore with the guilty feeling I have developed because of not being able to have sex. I am about to develop a complex. Please help me. I will be very happy if you could at least send me a guiding e-mail. I was raped when I was sixteen but as anal sex. Of course my husband doesn't know this; he is kind of narrow-minded. It had hurt so much that I have never felt such great pain ever since. After that day, I began having great fear. And now, whenever we try intercourse with my husband, everything goes normal during foreplay and I always tell myself that it will happen this time. I want him, I want to be with him, but when we come to that point, I start getting scared, sweating and contracting unwillingly, and I panic. Please help me. Otherwise I'll lose my husband…

A: As seen in your message, a sexual trauma experienced in the past does not allow the penis-vagina coupling due to the *principle of the subconscious attributing the past event to your husband*, no matter how much you love him. We are ready to do whatever we can to help you. Don't be afraid, you will not lose your husband and you will experience a happy relationship and togetherness. And don't feel guilty; with therapy, you will learn this natural process that you need to live as a woman, and you will experience sex in all aspects…

Q: We spoke on the phone earlier but I am writing you this e-mail in order to explain my situation in more detail and also to find out whether I am suitable for hypnosis, and also to learn if hypnosis is a method that will cure my problem. I have been married for exactly one year; yesterday was our first anniversary. I have been facing a vaginismus problem since the first days of our marriage. We had decided to leave it to time but unfortunately nothing got better. Later, after about six months, I decided to get professional help. I went to a recommended university professor who was an expert in his field. The treatment program he gave me consisted of anatomic knowledge of the vagina, sexual abstinence, exercises for the couple to learn about each other's bodies (Where sex and touching these areas were not allowed), Kegel Exercises and finally finger exercises... Frankly, I did not follow the doctor's program so much, but actually, the exercises were not so useful because my problem is primarily psychological. After trying the finger exercises for a couple of times, I could not do them because I felt nausea and a horrible discomfort. So I stopped seeing the psychiatrist after that stage. Because despite the fact that my doctor had asked for a strict sexual abstinence, I trial intercourse and failed once again... When I evaluate the passing year, I see that the solution for my problem lies in my acceptance of that area being filled with something and that there is nothing wrong with its presence, and that I will not feel pain. But unfortunately, I can't manage this. There has not been a serious sexual molestation or abuse in my past, but I think the fact that my family raised me like a boy during my sexual development period could have some effect. If I need to give an example, in order to keep me away from boys, my mother used to have possessive, protective suggestions like, "My daughter will not get married." I always perceived sexuality as disgraceful, harmful, etc. during my teenage years. Other than this, there is another thing that I experienced. When I was about thirteen or fourteen, I had witnessed a sexual intercourse. I was very frightened; I had thought that what the woman was going through was torturous, and I hadn't been able to get over it for a week... I guess that could have had an effect too.

Now I've told you my entire story, doctor. I am undecided between a psychiatrist's treatment and hypnosis. I don't know which one is suitable for me. As a matter of fact, I took an appointment at the sex disorders unit but as I said, I am so undecided... Because I can't tolerate another feeling of disappointment. Please let me know if you can really help me. Unfortunately, this illness has become very open to abuse in Turkey, due to the society's insensibleness and taboos. I was very curious about the methods of people who said they provided solution in a single session. I first read about it on your web site; it is very interesting that they give an injection and send people home, saying that they are cured! Finally, what do you have to say when you compare cognitive behaviorist treatment and hypnosis? I await your e-mail. Thank you very much, good luck in your work...

A: Your mail was caught in my mail filter; I just realized it today. I made sure our future communications will be all right. And I also added you into the vaginismus group. Now you can log in and check previous mails with your

Yahoo e-mail address. You will find most of the answers to your problem and to your questions on the web site and in the group messages.

From what you have written, there are subconscious negative espousals. You say you went to a professor, he gave you the homework and the things to do, but you could not progress even an inch. Behaviorist and cognitive approaches may be advised singularly or together, but when subconscious dynamics are in question, I advise you the cognitive, behaviorist and hypnotherapy method for removing your mental sets.

As you will see on our site, our method has been explained with all clarity and our cases have been shared without hesitation. There were so many wrong applications that we wanted to at least shed some light. We don't solve with hypnosis! Hypnosis could also be deficient in treatment on its own. Together with hypnosis, we apply a *therapy that includes behaviorist, cognitive, dynamic and existentialist approaches.* Finally, we advise you to choose the therapy that you believe in, trust and feel comfortable with.

Q: Hello, I am married for eight years. I am twenty-seven years old now. I have a vaginismus problem. We are having problems with my husband because of this and other reasons. At first, he did not accept treatment and just accused me. Later, I found out that such a problem existed and I was happy that I was not alone in this. My husband didn't support me; I was left alone with my problem. I couldn't tell anyone else about my problem. But before I had heard about it, I was thinking that it was psychological. And I told my husband. But he said that it was ridiculous, that a psychiatrist would be useless. In his defense, he was patient in his own way (Of course I gave him his due) but I also wanted him to understand me. We were unable to solve our problem. We drifted apart with each passing day. We couldn't come up with a solution. My efforts to see a doctor together were in vain. We were having sex somehow. Of course there were times when I felt pleasure. But I wanted to have a more sensual sex with longer lasting foreplay. But that would not happen. I was bothered by the fact that he was focused only on that point. But he believed he could solve the problem that way. I only had pleasure when he touched my genitalia. I was having orgasms.

I did not experience any sexual abuse or anything in the past. But I was even being greatly affected even by hearing about it, and I was thinking of intercourse as a very difficult thing. I mean, that was what I had heard from my surroundings in the past. The last time I went to a psychologist was three years ago. I had a meeting and after a few sessions, my husband came with me and we never went again, we didn't continue. During this treatment process, the doctor gave me antidepressants and I used them. He suggested finger exercises and I managed those too. I mean, I was able to do it with my finger. I saw that it could be, that it was not impossible. But I was feeling the same things during intercourse and we couldn't make it. I had been to a gynecologist for examination before the psychiatrist; there were no physical problems. We were not able to seek treatment in a major city because of my husband's and my busy work schedules. My husband wasn't so keen on it either. Our problem is ongoing and our marriage is coming to an end; it has been worn out quite a lot and we have reached an irreparable point. But I still wanted to write to you anyway. What can I do?

A: Vaginismus is not just the woman's problem. Yes, the woman does it with subconscious reflexes but she wants to have sex on the conscious level. When faced with situations like this, men need to help their wives at every step. It is essential that they go to therapy together, and listen to the physician's advice together. Easy and quick solutions may be found for the problem with the cooperation of the physician and the couple. From what you've written; you have left your therapy unfinished. But you have made progress. Only your subconscious fears are left. Even if your psychiatrist has prescribed antidepressants, we don't advise them so much because they reduce sexual desire in the long term. Instead of giving antidepressants, it seems much more rational to mentally work on the fears one by one and to win the fight in the battlefield. At times, the subconscious can nullify even the strongest of medicine. Intercourse may not be experienced despite epidural anesthesia or botox. Besides, these may not be enough, as seen in your case. Please talk to your husband once again and ask him to share this problem. Restart therapy together with your husband standing by you without being ashamed or bothered. Walk confidently to the solution…

Q: I too, have fears and distress during intercourse. I feel as if I would be deflowered even without having sex. But I have a son. And I had the child just so that we would not have intercourse for a year or two. I still have that fear. Now the fear of getting impregnated has been added to it. What am I to do?

A: Quite many consultees who apply to us for vaginismus say that they want to get pregnant somehow, just to be relieved from the pressure from their environment. But as you can see, ignoring vaginismus and somehow having a child does not bring a solution to the problem. The fears that remain in the subconscious, which we keep talking about, never leave you alone. It is as if there is a dragon with seven heads inside you and it rules over you. Therefore, the reasons need to be investigated with a good formulation and a *Cognitive + Behaviorist + Hypnotherapeutic* approach, and then a step-by-step battle must be given with the reasons in order to help you overcome your inner anxieties and fears. All seven heads of the dragon need to be destroyed. ☺

Q: I have been using XXX 50mg for a year. I was under a physician's supervision. First we increased the medicine to 100mg and now to 150mg. My question is; can I be cured with this medicine treatment? Or if the drugs don't provide a solution, would it be possible for me to be healed with hypnotherapy? Will drugs be necessary after this treatment? I mean, would there be a risk of starting drugs again?

A: The drug you are using is used in depression treatment and obsessive-compulsive disorders. If you have problems touching your genitals or if you have an obsession about hygiene (Like washing your hands a lot) in addition to vaginismus, the medicine you are taking could be supplementary. But no medicine can singlehandedly remove the fears nested in the subconscious, or the contractions. On the contrary, the subconscious is able to nullify medicine at times. Since I don't have enough information about you, I cannot say much on whether you can be cured or not. But most of the time, medicine treatment on its own remains deficient. Still, there could be variations between individuals. As mentioned in my early messages, hypnotherapy provides mental solutions. Even if we use vaginal dilatators for short terms with the cognitive and behaviorist approach, hypnotherapy provides great contribution to the solution. It could be disheartening for you in the future to hope that medicine alone can provide cure for vaginismus.

Q: My physician gave me finger exercises and prohibited us from trying intercourse. What is the logic behind this; shouldn't I try it when I feel confident in myself?

A: Even if you build up your self-confidence, do not skip any steps before it is the right time or before your physician suggests it. Can a child walk before crawling? The logic system behind could be listed as; first being able to do your finger exercises comfortably, then gaining your self-confidence and also building up your sexual desire during this process.

Q: Although I have been following the e-mails, I hadn't been able to write for a long time. As you know, my vaginismus problem is going on although I am pregnant. I've been seeing a psychologist for almost a month. He gives me the finger exercises that we all know. I am at the stage of trying it with two fingers, and then with my husband's finger. Today, my physician said that I could not have a normal delivery if I didn't overcome my problem, and that my baby would have to be taken with caesarean section. (Is this possible?) He also said, "You can't bring anything out, just like you can't take anything in." Frankly, I am very upset with this. I don't want days to pass. What will happen if I can't solve it until then? I am unbelievably stressed out right now. What do I need to tell to myself to speed things up, doctor? What kinds of suggestions should I be giving myself? I'm happy to talk to you again. I wish speedy recovery for all...

A: According to my knowledge and experience, a vaginismus problem doesn't create a caesarean indication. Because different hormones and mechanisms step in during labor, and the vagina expands to about four inches from which a baby's head can pass through. An approach suggesting that you can't get anything out if you can't get anything in, is good for nothing but to scare and intimidate you. This is not a correct approach for a sensitive vaginismus woman. But, your physician will want to perform vaginal examinations frequently before delivery. If you have contractions during examination and if you don't allow yourself to be examined, your physician will justifiably suggest caesarean for you.

Q: My physician had diagnosed me with this illness many years before, I mean about four years ago. I started treatment at a Medical Faculty, continued the sessions but at the time, we were just lovers with the person I am married to today so I couldn't do the exercises because we couldn't get together a lot. But I made my doctor think that I was. But I was able to manage one finger with the exercises they call Kegel. Then I got married. Now I am married for one month and still a vaginismus patient. I know the Kegel Exercises but I don't want to do them; yet, I still want this illness to go away. It always feels like it will heal on its own but we fail in every trial, and we aren't trying any more. I don't trust Kegel Exercises, like even that feels like it will hurt. I don't know what I need to do. I am one-month married but unhappy...

A: First of all, you have tried to mislead your physician during the times you took therapy, and as you can see, you have been the one who has failed. During therapy, never say things that are different than the ones you truly experience, or never act as if you have done the things that you actually have not... Honesty, trust and belief are the corner stones of therapy. We have applications that are different from the existing therapy concepts. We don't suggest Kegel Exercises. I think the Kegel Exercises you mention in your letter are the finger exercises. As seen in your case, the vaginismus woman can develop resistance against these, too. They may be rejected because they are perceived as homework or because of reservations. Or the couple is stuck at the penis stage following the finger stage. So, what do we do? We increase your mental capability under hypnosis, increase your belief, and forestall the contractions, pain, ache and fear. And our short-term triple feedback exercises for the vagina are usually done by our patients easily after the suggestions. As you are newly wed, my advice for now is to give yourself a two-month time period. Go over the things your previous physician had told you and apply them in order. You can reach me and get support at times when you are having problems. Don't exaggerate this situation you are in and don't remain unhappy; there are no vaginismus patients that have not been able to succeed with the right support. You will have ups and downs. But nothing will fall from the sky to heal you. You need to put in the effort…

Q: First, I'd like to thank you for your thoughts. Perhaps I'm just tired of trying and failing for four years. Before, I was asking myself if I had the taboo of not having sex before marriage, apparently it was not so. I make my husband and myself unhappy, and I don't have the right to. I'm thinking of starting today but believe me; I'm still worried about the pain. Do you think I could have results if I start at this stage?

A: Start by not blaming yourself anymore and without making yourself unhappy. Pain…but how much pain? Do you that a way of providing desensitization against pain is to come down on it step by step and to increase the pain tolerance. Stop at the point you feel pain. In the next trial, try to pass that step just a little bit and feel the pain at that new point, if there is any. And then another step… Before you know it, the penis will be inside the vagina after a serious effort… And no more pain!

Q: I am not receiving therapy. I am being treated by a gynecologist. I started directly with finger exercises and I managed them in a short time, like one week. You said that admission exercises that are gradually getting bigger are necessary, but it seems impossible to me because my hymen is intact. From what I know, only one finger can pass through the hymen gap. That is why I think I won't be able to go further with these exercises.

A: It is very hard to accept the term *impossible* in vaginismus. They used to say that 100 meter runners would never go under 14 seconds… 13sec, 12sec,

10sec, and now I think it is under nine seconds... We create impossibilities in our mind and then we believe them. ☺ But as you see that obstacles are overcome, that other women succeed in this, the belief of failure in our mind changes to success. This is actually one of the goals of this group, first of its kind in Turkey. To show you that you can do it. You are individuals with vaginismus and also teachers who educate each other. You are those who actually meet the problems and who apply the solutions, ones who are in pain and also in tears of joy. That is why you are so precious for each other...

"Look, if I placed a 30-foot long and 24-inch wide wooden plank in front of you and asked you to walk on it, I guess all of you would walk with your eyes open or closed. If I put that plank between two ridges at 65 feet high, you could not dare to walk. What has changed? You had walked on the same plank, even blindfolded... What have changed are the emotional factors and meanings you have ascribed to the events." So, want it, imagine a different moment, and do it! Are you too weak to succeed? No, you are very strong; think of the energy you spend during your contractions in every failed trial. You can do it...

Q: Hello Mr. Murat. Thank you for replying my message so quickly. I always read the incoming mails and I see that there are a lot of fellows in our situation. As a man, I love my wife very much. I can't think of a life without her and I will never allow such a thing to ruin our lives. As I said, it has been two and a half years since we got married and my wife worries herself a lot. Just out of her love for me, she thinks that I am unhappy, that I'll get fed up one day and that I will cheat on her. But I love her so much that if her life depended on my death, I wouldn't think for a split second to give my life for her. But we are unable to face our families because we still haven't been able to have intercourse and because she is still a virgin. I would like to come to see you but you are far away and also my job doesn't allow me. Please help us in this virtual platform. I read your mails; could you advise us any medicine or exercises? Thank you very much and best regards...

A: I hope that your care and love for your wife continues for a lifetime. It is a wanted, desired approach. You need to ignore the pressure from your families. More so because you are newly married. If only this could go away by suggesting a medicine or two, but that is mostly not possible. You will need to put in the work. Apply my suggestions in the group. Let your wife read the mails, too. Tell me what you are doing and I will support you whenever you are stuck...

Q: Doctor, there is something I don't understand. I do the finger exercises and one day it is so easy that I don't feel any contractions, but the next time (even if it is the next day) I have contractions again as if I have never exercised. I couldn't solve this problem. Isn't the whole point of the exercise being able to go further each time? Sometimes it happens in the opposite direction for me.

A: There is a situation that I often point out but that you are missing. If the reason of the vaginismus is a factor in the subconscious, you will experience such tides. As seen in the mail of a consultee that I have posted in the group yesterday, she had had botox twice and she has been receiving behaviorist therapy for a year but she cannot succeed. So, the therapy method needs to be changed. The treatment to be chosen must be one which does not obstinate with the subconscious but which rubs it the right way and which can change it in time. And one of such treatment methods is hypnotherapy. But it should a hypnotherapy with an active approach that is specific for the individual. Whenever you fight with the subconscious, it will win; never forget that. That is why it is essential to conform to the subconscious without obstinance. Our consultees, to whom we have provided remote education and who have performed the exercises we have given them at home on their own, are SIMPLE VAGINISMUS patients… I guess this is the group that can actually be cured by those who claim to heal in a single session. When you give appropriate exercises to such consultees and when you provide an ego-supporting approach, success will follow. Unfortunately, most of the vaginismus cases seen in Turkey are the types with interactions at the subconscious level. And a personalized *Cognitive + Behaviorist + Hypnotherapeutic* approach is appropriate.

Q: This is hard until you get over it, I guess. Once you do, maybe it will be a week before you even forget having such a problem. But those who experience it are still struggling inside that vortex. I have been having classical treatment for a month. I've come quite a way; even I am surprised with the distance I have covered with finger exercises. But I guess I will not be able to believe that I can do it until the final day. Vaginismus is like learning to swim, to ride a bicycle. Once you gather your courage and hit the pedals, you are able to do it after seeing that you don't fall, that you speed up. But there, we need wind to revive this belief. The air feels so droughty nowadays… There is no more wind from my right or from my left… What I'm trying to say is that I am solving the problem mechanically, yes, but I have been feeling very bad for the last week because I am in depression. I just don't want to talk to anyone, I just want to stay in my room and sleep. I eat only enough to keep me alive, I keep on trying to slur life over. For some reason, I feel that it is too late for the successes I have achieved to make me happy. There is a meaningless weariness over me. I stir up trouble for no reason and I cry, I upset my husband and torture myself too. I am even surprised if the meal I cook tastes nice.

You know the story of the ugly duckling…I feel exactly like the ugly duck there. I am about to give up on life. I have lost my health too, I can't sleep, I can't concentrate on work. I am always depressed all the time… People around me keep asking what is bothering me nowadays. How could I tell them? What would happen if I did? I keep asking why this is happening to me. And as I do, I start digging out the past. My old boyfriends… I went through my past with a fine comb. I wondered if one of them did this to me; such silly thoughts I have… I stood up today for just half an hour. I have formed five sentences at most. I am so unhappy I just can't explain, so unhappy…

A: As the treatment duration is prolonged, the patient has gotten into a psychological breakdown… Perhaps her physician will see her situation during the next session and start antidepressants! The medicine will heal the emotional state but it will reduce sexual desire and she will get into a complete viscous circle. The mechanical system and approach applied to this patient is at the verge of collapse… With this case, we observe the emotional meltdown created in the person with the applications which try to solve the problem only mechanically and which predominantly apply behaviorist therapies. With hypnosis and hypnotherapy, the patient's motivation is always kept high. Hypnosis and hypnotherapy shed light to your spiritual world. Behaviorist methods on their own will evaluate you as a mechanical piece… No matter what, Mrs. X, always remember that victory comes by standing up again after each defeat…

Q: Mr. Murat, I wanted to write to you because I am feeling terrible. I am a member who has been trying to convince her husband for treatment on this matter but who has failed. And I guess it is not necessary anymore because we are getting divorced. It's very difficult to write about this but this is the case. I've been reading all your letters but I couldn't succeed. My husband has stopped talking about this for a while but there have been other problems between us. We drifted apart each day, we began arguing more and more, and we have exhausted our respect to one another. I never wanted anything like this to happen but I couldn't help it. I was unable to do it, I tried a lot but it just wouldn't happen… It is our wedding anniversary on the 26th of this month but I guess we won't be celebrating it. We couldn't do it with my husband; I admit that. But I don't accept losing to vaginismus. I don't know what will happen in the coming days but he told me he would leave me. I haven't given up so I reached out to you and I believe I will overcome this thing called vaginismus. My family doesn't know about this… It's great to be a member of your web site; I hope I will read these messages as someone who has become a woman. In any case, I thank you very much. Good luck with your work…

A: You really need a guiding friend right now and you don't actually know what you are going to do. Your husband may say you will get divorced but there is an old saying, "Don't count the chicken before they hatch." You truly love him and maybe you are cursing your vaginismus. The wind of separation may die down until the 26th; words may have been said with anger. Besides, things don't happen so quickly when you say you will get separated, they take a lot of time. There will be opportunities for both sides to rethink. But despite everything, don't worry if you husband leaves you because of vaginismus. Let him stew in his own juice… Actually, he is showing his love for you with this decision he has made. He will leave you because of your vaginismus today, and tomorrow he will take a much harder hit from the person he marries afterwards, or he will be dumped because of falling into a situation such as yours… Or you may find another spouse that will make you much happier… The universe is founded in a complete harmony and balance. *If a butterfly flaps its wings in China, it could turn into a hurricane in America.* Just don't lose your belief and love for life, please. Maintain your respect toward your husband and to yourself. Each event we face has a meaning. Even if we cannot solve it at the time, every cloud has a silver lining. Do you know the story of Moses and the Prophet Khidr? It is in the Surah Al-Kahf. Could you please read the mentioned surah, verses from 60 to 82?

Everything we come across in life has a meaning… Something that looks good may harm us in the future, or some event that we see as evil may open a path for us toward goodness. (On this issue, I suggest that you read the story of Musa meeting Khidr.) Mrs. X, please be patient…

Q: Good night, Mr. Murat. I found out about your website while doing research, trying to find out what my problem was. After reviewing, I came to the conclusion that you could actually help me. I have been married for about fifteen months. I am twenty-five years old, I am a Taurus woman, I have a vaginismus problem, and on top it, I am four and a half months pregnant. The early times of my marriage went by with me trying to understand what my problem was. Even though I received professional help later, I was not successful. I was able to do the finger exercises given by my psychiatrist. But I was stuck at the two-finger exercise when my doctor went on vacation. So I'm also on a kind of holiday, too. Now, albeit rarely, we are trying penis penetration but I can't manage that. I want to tell you about my current and general mood. I had an arranged marriage with my husband. At first, I was not really into him and I thought that this was the reason and I told him I needed time. Nowadays, I love my husband, he's a perfect guy, both materially and morally, but it just doesn't happen. So the problem is somewhere else! I have always refrained from sex. I don't know why but I'd always felt like it is not such a pleasant thing (Unfortunately I still think so because of my pain and distress). I feel repulsed when the fluid from my husband (semen) touches my skin. Even looking at the penis disgusts me, let alone touching it. How pitiful, right? Of course, in such a situation, I am not able to control myself like my doctor asks me to, and allow penetration. As a matter of fact, I am trying to overcome this recently. I touched it a few times and I even made entrance trials under my control but I did that without touching with my hand, using a handkerchief. It makes me feel really sad and ashamed to write all this but I am ready for anything to be cured. Not for myself, but I want this mostly for my baby and for my husband. My current situation is that I can only allow it to touch the entrance of my vagina. When he tries to move forward, my contractions and distress begin. And this initiates a night with anger and stress. I still can't dare to do it. I also have lack of sexual drive and I can say that I am not affected by anything. Maybe this is causing most of the problem… I intend to do it every night but I just can't gather the courage. I have a personality that doesn't tolerate hardship or pain, and this makes it even more difficult for me. As I am so intolerant to pain, I can't even let a little penetration. I guess my greatest obstacle is fear! My husband is not here right now but when he comes home soon, he will look at me with hopeful eyes as if saying, "Could we do something tonight?" and he will meet my obstacles again and be very sad. This situation has worn out the both of us. So, where should I start in this case, doctor? I thank you in advance and hope speedy recovery to everyone…

A: You have repulsion, disgust, fear, and intolerance for pain and ache. As you can see, we can't just say vaginismus and move on. The thing is not just the finger exercises. The consultee has passed the finger exercises and she is stuck at the penis stage, and she has a complex structure. We don't know whether there has been an abuse in the past, but we think that there should be a cognitive or behaviorist structure that can explain her repulsion of semen and the penis tissue. This should be investigated and a multi-faceted supportive therapy needs to be applied. Our suggestion for this consultee is to stay in the group and follow the messages. All her questions will be answered whenever necessary. We think that this consultee needs to receive therapy directed toward her problems.

Q: Hello. I was just going to ask if vaginismus symptoms could be seen without trying intercourse. What I mean is, I haven't tried sexual intercourse yet but while receiving oral sex, at a certain stage, I involuntarily feel something I can't define, something like a cramp in my vagina. When I have this cramp-like thing in my vagina, I unwillingly stop my partner. I have never had an orgasm before. But I was familiar to this convulsion. I also used to feel this convulsion at my vagina at times when I need to go to the bathroom but can't go at that time, and when I am in a rush but can't get out of the house, and also during an erotic dream. All I have to do is to loosen myself up when the cramp comes but it's really hard. My question is; could it be vaginismus that is preventing me from having orgasms? I've never seen a problem like mine anywhere or heard it from anyone. Thanks in advance!

A: The cramp or convulsion you feel could just be trembling and contractions seen in some women who live orgasm at its peak. The fact that you experience the same thing during erotic dreams corroborates this idea. As for your question on whether it would cause vaginismus or if you have vaginismus, my suggestion is for you to use your finger or control rods made for this purpose to check your vagina entrance after getting married. You will find out whether it is a real contraction or not. As another cause, you could be experiencing a similar situation due to the effects of a sexual trauma from the past, or the effects of cognitive distortions on your behavior...

Q: Hello I am a twenty-four-year-old woman, married for five months. We could not have intercourse with my husband on our first night or on the following nights. I didn't have any fears or any dislike about this. The doctors said that my hymen is located high and that sexual intercourse would be difficult. We managed the first intercourse with difficulty, by using a local anesthetic drug. But after this, there have been no improvements in the following four months. I am still having very difficult, painful and torturous intercourses. Am I a patient that falls into the group you are treating? Or do you also think, like my other doctors, that mine is not a vaginismus problem? Thanks...

A: The fact that the hymen is thick, hard, more inverted than normal, being located higher, etc. do not necessarily prevent you from having intercourse. Such words may be said due to the necessity of basing the situation on an organic foundation. Still, it could be appropriate to see a few gynecologists and reevaluate after a hymen operation, if necessary. The word meaning of vaginismus is the involuntary contraction of the muscles at the lower part of the vagina. But other than this, fears, convulsions, the worry of feeling ache or pain, or as in your case, feeling great pain could hinder the intercourse. The important thing is to apply therapy to remove the contractions if there is ache or pain related to the contractions, and to avoid the torture you are feeling during sex.

Q: Hello, Mr. Murat. I have no problems with the finger exercises until I touch my hymen. As soon as I touch it, I can't go on, thinking that it will hurt. Wouldn't I be able to have an easier intercourse if my hymen was punctured by a gynecologist under anesthesia?

A: No, it would not. Why? You "don't want to continue thinking that it will hurt." You can see that the term *hurt* is in your mind, meaning that you have cognitive distortions. Or your pain threshold is low. Therefore, we don't advice the removal of the hymen. Let's say that you did remove it; the mechanical obstacle will have been removed but your problem will continue unless your cognitive frame of mind is changed.

Q: Hello X. I am going to ask a question to Mr. Murat based on your letter. Don't these lubricants, baby oil, vaseline, etc. cause any damage to the vagina tissue? After all, they all contain chemical substances.

A: That is correct; they are all chemical compositions. The vagina structure is made of mucosa, like the inside of the mouth. I don't advice it if the lubricants are oil-based; water-based ones could be preferred. If the amount of oil increases in the vagina, it could create fungus or other infections under the layer of fat.

Q: Dear Dr. Ulusoy, I am four-months married. We have been together with my wife for three years. We had sexual relationships during these three years but because of her sensitivity about the hymen, we have never tried a full intercourse. We failed in our trials during the first days of our marriage because of the extreme fear she was feeling. She didn't have any sexual aversions but she was straining herself a lot due to the fear she felt with the pressure of the penis, and she would just go cold. We were unable to overcome the problem on our own and we first consulted a gynecologist to see if there were any physical problems. During the examination, the gynecologist said that she didn't have a vaginismus problem but that her hymen was too thick and elastic, and that she could feel pain during sex because of this. And he offered to remove the hymen with a small operation. I agreed with him because when I examined my wife's hymen, I could notice that it was different from the other hymens I had seen in other sources. The operation was done and the obstacle was removed. Now we are able to have sexual intercourse; there are no vaginal contractions but her fears are still ongoing. The intercourse is very distressful and tense. She feels fear and pain. Although I tell her that we have a problem, she doesn't accept it. She says that she will get used to it and that her friends told her it would last for about a year. But I don't think it is normal at all because I can never get my penis in completely. The expression of pain and fear in her face causes me to lose my excitement, to lose my appetite and even to have erection problems. She used to have exaggerated thoughts about the hymen before getting married. She was saying that it would bleed a lot and that it would be difficult. In fact, one of her relatives had been sent back home because of not bleeding on her first night. My wife had told me that, ever since childhood, she used to check on herself every time she had the slightest difficulty (Like when she fell or rode a bike). Besides, she can't touch her vagina or allow anything like a finger, suppository or any other substance to enter. I know her problem is psychological but I don't know how to persuade her. In her view, there are no problems with our sex life because sex is already a painful thing, and only the hard-boiled (!) don't feel pain or fear.

A: I had posted a letter in the group earlier about the hymen being very thick and elastic. It could be thick but it would allow penetration if it is elastic. You might remember the mail from X in the group about this; gynecologists had used the same terms for her, too. Actually her letter is also on our web site. She could manage intercourse only after the removal of her contractions by hypnotherapy. Your problems are still going on after the removal of the hymen and she is having a hard time allowing the penis inside. I am curiously waiting to see when you and the physicians will stop messing with the hymen that is treated like a scapegoat. In your story, it is clearly apparent that fears from the past are preventing the relationship.

Q: Hello Mr. Murat, I am married for 21 months and I am 32 years old. Unfortunately, I too, am facing a vaginismus problem. I went to a gynecologist in the ninth month of our marriage and she applied finger exercises. At first, I couldn't do it at all. But I managed it after ten or fifteen days and I was very happy. Unfortunately we were not able to go any further and the treatment was left halfway. Right now, I don't have problems with the fingers but we can't do anything more. And this makes us really unhappy. There is always something missing in our lives. This problem is gnawing at my brain all the time. I don't know when or how we can solve this problem. I know that both the problem and the solution are in my mind but I just can't. Please help me! I don't have the possibility to be treated in another city because I am a working woman; what can I do?

A: Here, we see once again that being able to do the finger exercises doesn't mean that you will be able to have intercourse. This consultee has passed the finger phase but can't go on to the penis phase. At this point where you are stuck at, you need to continue with a therapy that will eliminate the problem.

Q: Mr. Murat, it's me again, X. Although I can't write so frequently, I am writing at times when I'm really depressed because I have no one else to talk to. We haven't been able to start treatment yet but as I said earlier, you are my only hope. Besides, other than this vaginismus problem, I have the fear of being alone in the house and it influences my life terribly, and I don't know if there is a connection between this and my fear of sex. There is something I want to ask you today before I come to see you. Is it possible to eliminate finger exercises in your treatment process? I mean, although I am so informed, thinking of it moves me away from everything, even from the hope of being cured. I assume this trauma reached such heights after the gynecologic examination. Otherwise I had tried it a little in the past and I had managed it, a little. My questions seems a bit silly after all this correspondence and after reading the mails of others in the group, but I am writing whatever is going through my mind, whatever I am feeling right now. As a matter of fact, I am at the brink of eruption but I don't have anybody to have a heart-to-heart talk. Anyway, I don't want to take too much of your time. I wish you a happy Eid. Bye…

A: First of all, good morning. Finger exercises are techniques used by the behaviorist method. Since we work on the problem with hypnotherapy first and enable to the body to loosen up, the homework we give become easier to do.

Q: Dear Dr. Murat, is it helpful or harmful to make the vaginismus woman watch pornographic movies or photographs? For instance, I downloaded photos of fisting and large penis penetration from the internet and showed them to my wife. She told me she was disgusted and I never did it again.

A: Oh boy, what have you done Mr. X ☺ As befits the name, pornography is far from aesthetics; they are movies, which heighten feelings of lust and in which only the animal instincts are at the forefront. When you made your wife, who already had fears, watch them, you created another trauma. Fisting and large penises… ☺ Now whenever the poor woman wants to try sex, she will think about them and her fear, her panic will increase even further. This is a true manifestation that you don't understand the vaginismus woman, your wife…

Q: Hello Murat (I hope you don't mind because I feel so sincere and close to you already). I had sent you an e-mail a few days ago, saying that I was doing finger exercises and that I was able to allow three fingers in but my vagina would not allow it at the penis stage. I had also mentioned the immense pain I felt and I had asked whether I was psychologically creating this pain. And you said that this was a fake, deceiving pain. This gave me a lot of courage and knowing this, I decided to try it. I was determined this time and I was going to do it. We started making love with my husband but we were both really tense. We just couldn't get aroused as we did in our previous lovemaking, and as the goal was different, we rushed for the penetration but it entered easily in our first try. In fact, I felt no pain but it was possible only when I was on top. My vagina didn't allow penetration when he came on top and then my husband said he didn't feel anything and his erection died. We tried to stimulate it later; he was having erections but it passed quickly. I began feeling pain in later trials. The pain gradually increased and finally it prevented entrance. But I forced it a lot and felt a lot of pain. Everything just went downhill and we both became alienated from sex.

I lied down the next day as if I was sick. I couldn't touch my vagina at all; it was hurting like it had been torn to pieces. I couldn't sit and I couldn't even touch my husband. Even just the thought of touching him reminds me of the pain. I don't ever want to have sex again in my life and I feel terrible, believe me. I still love my husband a lot but I feel like I'm losing my mind. Sex just reminds me of great pain and I feel like I am going to throw up. I don't know why it happened. Please tell me what I should do. I really want to come and see you but it is impossible for the time being. Has my problem gone worse or will these feelings pass?

A: Look, you are having this problem because of an emotional distortion and/or an underlying trauma. You had such a bad result because you made a trial before this was solved, before receiving therapy about it I mean. First of all, if you perceive something as homework and try to do it that way, of course there will be difficulties. Secondly, you beat your subconscious although that was so hard, or you thought you did. You managed it when you were on top. Okay, congratulations… Until now, we see how strong your willpower is. But whenever the conscious gets into a fight with the subconscious, it is always the subconscious and the defense mechanisms that win. As seen in your letter, it happened at first but then it gradually prevented penetration. Your husband's loss of erection is not a problem right now. It is a temporary situation and it could be overcome with temporary precautions. But you have been badly injured during the battle you had with your conscious mind. Now you have connected sex with pain, even the thought of touching your husband or of sex gives you pain. See, the important reaction is your *feeling as if you would throw up*. As the basis of the problem was not solved, the subconscious has developed defense systems to prevent intercourse. Actually it is shouting out to you, saying, "You have to solve the underlying problem…" It is communicating with you via your body. As for my reply on whether the problem has gone worse, I think not. But the conscious and the subconscious measured each other up and unfortunately you were badly affected. In this case, it seems inevitable for you to receive therapy…

SURVEY RESULTS

I. How many places did I apply to for my vaginismus problem? – 2011

Total number of participants:	4,849	
I did not receive treatment	3,201	(65%)
I went to one place, could not heal	823	(17%)
I went to at least three places, could not heal	327	(7%)
I went to at least five places, could not heal	82	(2%)
I went to five or more places, could not heal	170	(4%)
I went to one place, I was cured	149	(3%)
I went to more than one place, was cured	91	(2%)

Evaluation of the above survey as of March 2015

Total number of participants:	5,902	
I did not receive treatment	3,902	(66%)
I went to one place, could not heal	1,010	(17%)
I went to at least three places, could not heal	397	(7%)
I went to at least five places, could not heal	103	(2%)
I went to five or more places, could not heal	211	(4%)
I went to one place, I was cured	177	(3%)
I went to more than one place, was cured	102	(2%)

The results of the same survey at different times are almost identical. Although four years have passed, and despite the fact that the number of vaginismus therapists and sexual therapy trainings have increased, classical treatments still have an almost 30% failure rate. The patients are going from therapist to therapist like billiard balls. And this shows us that the existing and applied classical vaginismus treatments are not curative for the vaginismus seen in Turkey. It is for this reason that The Dr. Ulusoy Method, which comprises Cognitive Therapy + Behaviorist Therapy + Hypnotherapy, provides much better results when compared to classical treatments (Solely cognitive, solely behaviorist, or cognitive + behaviorist).

II. I can't have intercourse with my partner because

Total number of participants: 194

I have great fears like; it will hurt, it will bleed a lot, it will be ruptured, the penis is too big	141	(73%)
I have been sexually abused in the past	4	(2%)
My partner doesn't show me enough care or love	4	(3%)
I don't like sex and don't take clitoral pleasure	13	(7%)
I was raised with sexual prohibitions and protection	31	(15%)

III. For my vaginismus problem

Total number of participants: 930

I go to a gynecologist	135	(15%)
I go to an anesthesiologist	8	(1%)
I go to a psychiatrist	92	(10%)
I go to a psychologist	69	(7%)
I go to one who can solve it a single session	86	(9%)
I pay regard to gender while choosing a physician, I go to a female physician	31	(3%)
I go to a hodja because there is a spell	43	(5%)
I go to an experienced physician who works on Vaginismus and whom I trust	466	(%50)

CHAPTER 2

"DR. ULUSOY METHOD" IN VAGINISMUS TREATMENT

In this chapter, you will find the details of The Dr. Ulusoy Method in vaginismus treatment, as well as patients' comments. The Dr. Ulusoy Method is a treatment method that leads to solution in three phases and in an average of one and a half days. This method eclectically incorporates *Hypnotherapy + Cognitive Therapy + Behaviorist Therapy*. And in hypnotherapy, it utilizes "Dr. Ulusoy HIT" as the induction technique. This chapter is designed for therapists. It is also intended for informing vaginismus patients on our method.

AN ANECDOTE AND
THE CAKE METAPHOR

Over the years, you don't realize what you are doing in the actual moment. When you look back from the point you have reached, you are able to see the events better and you realize how the pieces of the puzzle fall into place.

In 2001, I opened my first private clinic and began working on hypnosis. By the end of the third year, in a period of time when I seriously considered closing my clinic and returning to my old job at the state hospital, I received a foreign guest, a professor. We talked about hypnosis. Before leaving, he said, "Doctor, Turkey and its people need you. Don't ever give up working on hypnosis. Then he took out an evil eye talisman and gave it to me, saying, "And here, this is customary for us. May it protect you from evil eyes."

I was very affected with these words and I decided not to close by business despite the hard conditions of both my job at the state and of my practice. It was very interesting that I received my first vaginismus patient in the following months. I did not have much knowledge about vaginismus. I knew from foreign literature that classical treatment had a structure that lasted for twelve weeks. Apart from this information, I tried to see my patient's problems. With my experience on hypnotherapy, we focused directly on her problems. And I reached a result in a very short time. Since then, I have been creating practical solutions and new definitions with the experiences I obtain from my patients.

We are petty subjects, we are unable to know what is good or bad for us. Each of us has a mission in life. When we voluntarily want to move away from this mission, we are somehow redirected to where we need to be. My childhood years went by with reading a lot, other than schoolbooks, and by making experiments at home. While in primary school, the daughter of my mother's teacher friend had brought me an applied experiment book. I had done the experiments in the book over and over again. Other than that, I had produced shampoos by melting soaps and adding perfume to it. I had also built simple electronic circuits according to their schemes. I had a vivid imagination even as a child. I would visualize things first and then I would make them. My curiosity was extremely high. Sometimes this could be very dangerous for me. As in sticking a nail into the plug socket, or as in finding yourself in the other corner of the room with a big explosion and a fireball after pouring gas oil on the cinder in the log burner that seemed to be put out...

So, how was The Dr. Ulusoy Method developed? Let me tell you about it by describing how a cake is baked...

The Cake Metaphor

Here is a memory of mine on curiosity and reaching results.

A well-risen cocoa cake that is soft, spongy and extremely palatable... The cakes I ate didn't have the taste I was looking for. Middle school years... At our summer house... I bought a lot of flour, sugar, eggs, vanillin, baking powder, milk, yoghurt and oil from the market. I was making a small tray of cake almost every other day. I first started with a recipe I knew. Then I thought about what I needed to change in order to reach the result I wanted, and I began using the ingredients at different ratios. I guess it had been about fifteen days when the homefolk and the neighbors had grown tired of eating cake. But I had reached the formula suiting my taste. Now I look back and think; the thing that lies under my reducing the treatment process duration to one and a half days by first using hypnotherapy on its own and then adding cognitive and behaviorist treatments to it, and then developing a hypnosis induction technique, is the fact that my mom and dad had supported me and allowed me to bake cakes every day without any restrictions...

2004 Tıbbi Hipnoz Kongresi – T.C. Yeditepe Üniversitesi

THE EFFECTS OF HYPNOTHERAPY IN A VAGINISMUS PHENOMENON

2004 Medical Hypnosis Congress – Yeditepe University, Dr. Murat Ulusoy

Summary

Vaginismus is virtually a conditioned reflex of the subconscious causing the contraction of the muscles surrounding the entrance of the vagina to prevent the penis from penetrating the vagina.

Keywords

Vaginismus, vaginismus treatment, vaginismus cure, hypnosis, hypnotherapy, psycho-hypnotherapy

Introduction and Aim

The case presentation is the treatment of a vaginismus case using the cognitive therapy and hypnotherapy in addition to the behaviorist therapy. The principle of the vaginismus treatment is not only to provide the entrance of the penis into the vagina just once, but for it to have a lifelong effect. It also aims to treat the individual's sexual desire and perception.

Material

A thirty-year old patient, married for three years to her beloved husband. At the beginning of the three-year marriage, despite having about four months of behaviorist therapy and medical treatment, she had not been able to manage finger exercises other than externally touching the genitalia, or to have penis-vagina intercourse. She was told during her gynecological examination that her hymen was thick and an operation was advised. But our consultee did not accept the operation. During the anamnesis, it was observed that she had vaginismus due to cognitive reasons.

Method

Classical hypnosis methods and a method that included behaviorist and cognitive applications by using Albrecht's three-word hypnosis induction were applied to this patient with vaginismus. Sessions were planned as weekly meetings.

Sessions

Session 1: Hypnosis was explained, her questions about hypnosis were clarified and her worry especially on loss of consciousness was eliminated. Deep trance was obtained. After the first session ended, she was asked, "What do you think hypnosis is?" to which she replied, "It is the loss of body control." She was then provided with the suggestion that, just as her body could go out of her control, each muscle group could also be taken under control individually.

Session 2: She said that she had been able to do the finger exercises easily after the first session. But she was having the fear of feeling pain.

Age regression was performed. She remembered that in her primary school years, a relative of hers had touched her from behind while she was sleeping and he had ejaculated on her, and that she had woken up in fear. Abreaction occurred and she began crying. She was encouraged to cry. Suggestions were given to help her get rid of the negative emotional burden of the event. Her peace with the past was provided. She was supported for not feeling grudges, anger or rage.

Session 3: She was more self-assured when she came and her focus on success was observed. Glove anesthesia was applied. The pain-free area created on her hand was transferred to her vagina and its surroundings. She was taught how to transfer of the anesthetic area with a post-hypnotic keyword.

Session 4: She said that her fear, anxiety, withdrawal and worry of feeling pain were reduced very much during their intercourse trials. It was learned that the penis was able to penetrate an inch. Suggestions were given to her on the perception of the penis as part of the body.

She was taken into trance with Albrecht's three-word induction. As the symbol of the problem, she saw a bright black bug, and as the symbol of inner source, she saw a white four-leaf clover. She was asked to visualize the solution symbol during intercourse.

Session 5: Despite the fact that the patient was very relaxed and that she said she was ready for intercourse, she informed us that her husband had developed a secondary erection problem during the passing week and that they were unable to have the experience. (Seesaw Effect.)

Levitra 10mg was offered for the man's erectile problem. The patient was taken into trance again. She was given suggestions on taking pleasure during the experiences she would have and during intercourse. She felt the experience with visualizations (Simulation Technique). Toward the end of the session, she was asked to visualize the solution symbol again, and each leaf of the clover was matched with a suggestion as below.

Leaf 1: Relaxation
Leaf 2: Pleasure
Leaf 3: Removal of ache and pain
Leaf 4: Taking pleasure in repeating intercourses and easily managing the penis-vagina relationship

Findings

A total of five sessions were carried out. Progress was obtained after each session. The vaginismus problem was solved after the fifth session.

Discussion

Behaviorist and cognitive methods are used in vaginismus treatment. It has been observed that the application of the behaviorist and cognitive methods under trance increases effectiveness.

Result

The patient's existing complaints were removed with the application of classical hypnosis, Albrecht's three-word hypnosis, behaviorist and cognitive methods, and visualization. It is thought that the application has been more effective than traditional methods for vaginismus treatment. It would be more appropriate to work with multiple cases, rather than one.

1. Cognitive factors for our patient
   a. Sees sexuality as a taboo
   b. Is repulsed by sex
   c. Doesn't like to look at, to touch or be touched by the penis
   d. Feels insecurity toward her husband, thinks that he will abandon her if she lets him enter her body (Abandonment anxiety)
   e. Has fear of feeling pain during intercourse, displays contraction at the legs, withdrawal and pushes her husband away
   f. Cannot touch her genital area
   g. As a pleasant nuance, was raised with the suggestion of her mother while she was a child, "There is a blue bead between your legs; it will fall if you open them."
2. Seesaw Effect: The erection problem, which can be seen in men during the treatment process of vaginismus patients, has been named the *Seesaw Effect* by Dr. Murat Ulusoy.
3. Simulation Technique: The technique of making the patient experience a comfortable relationship under trance by visualization and within the desire-seduction-orgasm trio, is named the *Simulation Technique* by Dr. Murat Ulusoy.

Sources

1. *The Gate to the Resurrection of Reality, Hypnosis, Volume 1*, Dr. Tahir Özakkaş, Özak Publishing House, Second Edition, 1993 Kayseri
2. *The Gate to the Resurrection of Reality, Hypnosis, Volume 2*, Dr. Tahir Özakkaş, Özak Publishing House, First Edition, 1995 Kayseri
3. *Hypnotherapy in Sexual Problems*, Dr. Tahir Özakkaş, Özak Publishing House, First Edition, 1993 Kayseri
4. *Practicing Cognitive Therapy: A Guide to Intervent*, Robert L. Leahy, Translated by: Hasan Hacak - Muhittin Macit - Ferruh Özpilavcı, Litera Publishing, First Edition, 2004, İstanbul
5. *Cognitive Therapy and Emotional Disorders*, Aaron T. Beck, MD, Translated by: Aysun Türkcan, Litera Publishing, First Edition, 2005 İstanbul
6. *Holistic Psychotherapy*, Dr. Tahir Özakkaş, Litera Publishing, Second Edition, 2004, Istanbul

Note: This case that I presented during the 2006 Hypnosis Congress contains the treatment method that I applied during those years. And in the 2011 congress, I presented *The Dr. Ulusoy Method for vaginismus treatment that provides solution in three phases and in an average of one and a half days.*

THE EFFECT OF MAYALAMA[3] IN VAGINISMUS TREATMENT

Medical Hypnosis Congress – 2005, Yeditepe University
Dr. Murat ULUSOY

Summary

Vaginismus is virtually a conditioned reflex of the subconscious causing the contraction of the muscles surrounding the entrance of the vagina to prevent the penis from penetrating the vagina (The Merck Manual).

Keywords

Vaginismus, vaginismus treatment, vaginismus cure, hypnosis, hypno-therapy, psycho-hypnotherapy, mayalama

Introduction and Aim

Patients were divided into two groups, one of which mayalama session was added at the beginning of the treatment, while in the other group, not added. In the comparison of the duration of the therapies, a statistically significant decrease in the group with mayalama session was observed. The principle of the vaginismus treatment is not only to provide the entrance of the penis into the vagina just once, but for it to have a lifelong effect. It also aims to treat the individual's sexual desire and perception.

Material

20 cases, who have applied for treatment between the years 2002 and 2006, whose ages ranged from 21 and 44, who were at least primary school gradu-ates, and have had vaginismus problems for a duration between two months and 14 years, were taken.

---

(3) In the 1950s, Dr. Hüsnü Ismet Öztürk had designated the first step of conscious hypnosis as "informing and taking consent of the patient" where he highlighted the importance of *the acceptance of the patient*. He called this MAYA (Making Acceptance with Your Awareness) and in Turkish it is used with the suffix "lama" which is similar to the "-tion" suffix in English. So, "Mayalama" means "Fermentation" in English, perfectly describing *preparing the patient for treatment*.

Method

Ten cases received hypnotherapy without mayalama, ten cases received hypnotherapy with mayalama.

Group 1 - The number of sessions during vaginismus treatment without mayalama

Case1...6 sessions	Case6...2 sessions
Case2...4 sessions	Case7...9 sessions
Case3...7 sessions	Case8...5 sessions
Case4...3 sessions	Case9...7 sessions
Case5...8 sessions	Case10...6 sessions

Group 2 - The number of sessions during vaginismus treatment with mayalama

Case1...3 sessions	Case6...3 sessions
Case2...4 sessions	Case7...5 sessions
Case3...2 sessions	Case8...2 sessions
Case4...3 sessions	Case9...3 sessions
Case5...5 sessions	Case10...4 sessions

Their vaginismus problems have been cured by providing penis-vagina relationship in at least two positions.

Findings

The average number of sessions in Group 1 needed for success: $57/10 = 5.7$
The average number of sessions in Group 2 needed for success: $34/10 = 3.4$

Discussion

When mayalama is performed in the hypnotherapy applied in addition to behaviorist and cognitive methods during vaginismus treatment, it has been observed that the number of sessions required for treatment has been significantly reduced when compared to the group that has not been provided with mayalama.

Result

It is thought that hypnotherapy applied with mayalama is also effective in reducing the number of sessions required for vaginismus treatment when compared to traditional methods.

Sources

1. *The Gate to the Resurrection of Reality, Hypnosis, Volume 1,* Dr. Tahir Özakkaş, Özak Publishing House, Second Edition, 1993 Kayseri
2. *The Gate to the Resurrection of Reality, Hypnosis, Volume 2,* Dr. Tahir Özakkaş, Özak Publishing House, First Edition, 1995 Kayseri
3. *Hypnotherapy in Sexual Problems,* Dr. Tahir Özakkaş, Özak Publishing House, First Edition, 1993 Kayseri
4. *Practicing Cognitive Therapy: A Guide to Intervent,* Robert L. Leahy, Translated by: Hasan Hacak - Muhittin Macit - Ferruh Özpilavcı, Litera Publishing, First Edition, 2004, İstanbul
5. Cognitive Therapy and Emotional Disorders, Aaron T. Beck, MD, Translated by: Aysun Türkcan, Litera Publishing, First edition, 2005 İstanbul
6. *Holistic Psychotherapy,* Dr. Tahir Özakkaş, Litera Publishing, Second Edition, 2004, Istanbul
7. Ali Eşref Müzezzinoğlu, *Conscious Hypnosis* book series and Mayalama CDs
8. Dr. Hüsnü Öztürk, *Hypnosis and Mayalama* CDs

DR. ULUSOY'S CONTRIBUTIONS TO VAGINISMUS TREATMENT AND DEFINITIONS

Based on years of hypnosis and hypnotherapy research, and case experiences, I try to continue breaking new grounds in vaginismus treatment.

1. The method we apply in therapy is *The Dr. Ulusoy Method* which contains an individual holistic psychotherapy approach and which emphasizes on vaginismus-specific hypnotherapy techniques.

2. I have made a case poster presentation on the effectiveness of hypnotherapy in vaginismus treatment at the 1ˢᵗ Medical Hypnosis Congress in 2004 with local and foreign attendance.

3. During the 2ⁿᵈ Medical Hypnosis Congress in 2005, I declared that the secondary erection problem that may be seen in men during vaginismus treatment has been named as the **Seesaw Effect – Dr. Ulusoy**, and that the visualization that is performed as the final step of the treatment has been named the **Simulation Technique – Dr. Ulusoy**.

4. At the 3ʳᵈ Medical Hypnosis Congress I declared that the average number of sessions has been reduced to 3.6 by using the *Mayalama Technique.*

5. In vaginismus cases, after the passing of a certain time with only foreplay and no intercourse, the woman gets used to the notion that intercourse will not happen after foreplay so she feels relatively more comfortable. We call this **Relative Relaxation – Dr. Ulusoy.**

6. In the 65 case studies between January 2008 and May 2008, I added the *Intensified Attack Treatment and the Lozanov Technique* and reduced the average treatment time to one and a half days.

7. I have adapted the imagination techniques of hypnosis to the problems

faced in vaginismus, and I have named it **NVP (Neuro Visual Programming) – Dr. Ulusoy** in 2008.

8. I have defined **The Classification of Vaginismus Patients – Dr. Ulusoy** in 2008.

Vaginismus Classification

i.   Those who cannot touch the labia majora or labia minora, or in between (Outer genitalia).

ii. Those who can touch the outer genital area but not inside the vagina.

iii. Those who can touch the outer genitalia and the vagina and can direct fingers inside, but who cannot have the penis experience.

iv. Those who are in one of the three groups mentioned above and who do not have contractions, but who cannot allow the penis inside (Those with hip problems, breathing control problems or with problems of transferring of authority).

v.   Those who are in one of the first three groups mentioned above and who have internal or external contractions ranging from minor to severe, and who cannot take in the penis.

As seen, various categories appear when we talk about vaginismus. Moreover the factors listed below also have effect on the woman at different proportions, so the vaginismus illness almost resembles an ivy.

1. The woman's own character patterns (i.e. panic attack, obsession, perfectionist structure, phobic and afraid of everything…).
2. Lack of sexual education and knowledge.
3. Physical differences between man and woman.
4. Cognitive, behavioral, dynamic and existentialistic factors.

Therefore, the vaginismus treatment should be planned by taking into consideration all these details.

9. **Intermittent Vaginismus,** which I have defined in 2008, describes the situation when couples, who receive deficient and/or irregular treatments, or who don't get treated but try to solve the problem on their own with finger exercises and intercourse trials, think that the problem is solved when they manage to have the penis head or half of the penis inside the vagina but still cannot have a comfortable intercourse. While they are able to cover ground in some of their trials, they are unable to have the experience in other trials due to fears and contractions. We observe that women can

become pregnant in intermittent vaginismus but that they are unable to make progress in terms of intercourse. In such cases, it is possible to see couples, married for two to fifteen years, who have children but who cannot have intercourse. They apply for treatment many years later in order to have a comfortable intercourse.

10. **Learned Vaginismus Affiliated with Experience (Behavioristic) – Dr. Ulusoy, 2009.**

a. Sometimes when couples are unable to have the first intercourse, the push themselves to go through with the intercourse. But vaginismus that originates from mental fears may get worse.

b. Or, while the woman has no problems, it could be considered as learned vaginismus if she is forced into intercourse by the man on the first night.

c. Or the projection of an experienced molestation would fall under the scope of this topic.

d. Learned Vaginismus with Stigmatization (Identification): The stories that the woman has heard from her environment about the difficulties of the first intercourse could trigger first night frights for healthy individuals like dominos tipping over one another. These are also called cognitive reasons.

11. **Learned Helplessness in Vaginismus - Dr. Ulusoy, 2009**
Couples that think the intercourse will happen by itself over the years leave the matter to time. And during this time period, they occasionally have failed experiences. As time goes by and as intercourse doesn't happen, the couples refrain from trying intercourse and at a further stage, they even avoid touching or making love to each other. We call this *Learned Helplessness in Vaginismus.*

12. Between the years 2005 and 2006, I provided online pro bono support to 146 vaginismus patients and helped them overcome their problems.

13. As presented at the 5th Medical Hypnosis Congress, I have **reduced the vaginismus treatment duration to one and a half days** on average per therapy with the three-stage Dr. Ulusoy Method which contains hypnotherapy techniques specific to vaginismus and which is a cognitive – behaviorist approach (2011).

14. The main factors that influence the course of vaginismus treatment, new descriptions and therapy options that I have defined.

- **The Princess Effect** (Dr. Ulusoy, 2009): This is seeing vaginal intercourse as a way of dominating the man, using it as a way of rewarding or punishing, and connecting her other desires in life and expectations from the man to sex (Existentialist approach, hypnotherapy)

- **The Blue-Eyed Girl Effect** (Dr. Ulusoy, 2009): We can also call this the *being the little girl of the family effect*. The woman resembles a fragile flower raised in a flowerpot. She is overly sensitive to pain (Touching the vagina). Burning, pressure and the feeling of bluntness are emotions she has a hard time getting used to. (Behaviorist approach, metaphors and suggestions)

- **Urine Incontinence Problem** (Dr. Ulusoy, 2009): This defines the habit of holding one's urine for eight, 12, 24 or 48 hours, whether connected to OCD (Obsessive Compulsive Disorder) or not. When this habit goes on for many years, the urinary bag cannot find any place to go in the front so it leans more to the back, onto the front vaginal wall. It is always problematic for something to penetrate into the vagina with such patients. They feel the pressure very intensely. They say that they feel as if they will have to urinate at any moment, that they may not be able to hold it. At the same time, they perceive an intense neurogenic and disturbing stimulus due to the fact that the urinary bag is rich with neural networks. (Behaviorist approach)

- **The Sympathetic Spouse Effect** (Dr. Ulusoy, 2009): The real understanding man is the spouse who realizes that this is an illness and that steps need to be taken for its treatment, and also who proves this by providing support during the treatment process. The opposite situation is a man who says, "Okay honey, don't you worry. Let's go," at times when a behaviorist approach is needed during treatment and when his spouse is having examination anxiety, or a man who hinders the treatment by remaining silent and accompanying his spouse's fear. (Persuasion)

- **Tree Theory** (Dr. Ulusoy, 2009): The main factors in the forming of vaginismus are not actually the cognitive, behaviorist, dynamic or existentialist factors. These are the branches and leaves of the tree. What creates the problem are the tree's trunk and roots. One of the sisters in a family with two or more sisters may have vaginismus while the other one(s) have comfortable relationships. When looking at the general characteristics of the vaginismus women, we observe that they have the feature of taking a negative view at every event in life. Despite the fact that they are able to see and experience what is right, their belief system hits bottom very quickly and focuses on inability and failure. (Even during the exercises, they focus on the empty side of the glass.) A father, working as a technical draftsman, sat down his daughter when she reached puberty and informed her on the genital organs and intercourse by drawing up the genital organs, but his daughter appeared before us as a vaginismus patient. So, this means that the main problem in vaginismus is the deficiency of supporting their self-confidence while raising our daughters. We can also call this the cowardice of moving forward against any situation she faces in life. (Persuasion, reorganizing the belief system, behaviorist approach, hypnotherapy)

- **The Psoas Muscles in Ethiology** (Dr. Ulusoy, 2018): It is not the pelvic floor muscles but the Psoas Muscles that play an active role in vaginismus. Control of Psoas Muscles is obtained with hypnosis and feedback-assisted examination, and Holotropic Breathwork.

- **Therapy Approach Options in Other Problems Faced in Vaginismus Treatment**
  o Bodily contractions originating from the mind (Hypnotherapy)
  o Sensitivity toward the vagina tissue (Cognitive - Behaviorist approach)
  o The sensitivity arising in the lower abdominal region when something enters the vagina (Cognitive – Behaviorist approach, persuasion)
  o Fear and anxiety of examination (Hypnotherapy, cognitive approach, persuasion)
  o Erectile dysfunction, other sexual desires and impulses of the man such as fetishism (Medical approach, hypnotherapy, sex education)
  o Quarrels and fight among couples (Short term family therapy)
  o Thoughts of failure (Providing positive belief system)
  o Hymen deformation, bleeding and the related pain (Medical approach)
  o Different and negative treatments tried in the past (Providing belief of success, persuasion)
  o OCD, panic attack, conversive episodes, refraining from intercourse, flight due to fear or panic, nausea and vomiting (Cognitive approach, hypnotherapy)
  o Molestation or rape experienced in the past (Hypnotherapy)
  o Sexual oppression by the family (Hypnotherapy)
  o Cognitive distortions (Hypnotherapy)
  o Increasing the patient's capability to carry out homework (Hypnotherapy)
  o Allowing the spouse to resume control in the penis experience and in the behaviorist approach (Cognitive approach, hypnotherapy, indirect suggestions)
  o Penis circumference being larger than normal. Penis-vagina incompatibility in cases of narrow vagina and large penis (Behaviorist approach)
  o Cultural coding; not accepting examination by a male physician. (Per-

suasion; the physician's competence and therapy success rate is more important than gender.)

15. At the 12th ESH (European Society of Hypnosis) Congress of Hypnosis in 2011, I shared my retrospective analysis and survey results for 450 cases in addition to my presentation which included The Dr. **Ulusoy Hypnosis Induction Technique** and **Dr. Ulusoy Vaginismus Treatment Method.**

16. At the 1st Anatolian Neuroscience and Sexual Health Congress in 2015, I presented **The Dr. Ulusoy Method for Vaginismus Treatment** and **The Five-Step Gate Model** (5-BK – Dr. Ulusoy) that was restructured for psychiatrists and psychologists.

VAGINISMUS
TREATMENT FORMULA

(Dr. Ulusoy 2011)

A (ab) + B (cdef) + C (ghij) = Solving of the problem, experiencing intercourse

Main Factors

A: Dr. Ulusoy HIT (Hypnosis Induction Technique) and VTM (Dr. Ulusoy Vaginismus Treatment Method which is a cognitive, behaviorist, dynamic and existentialist formulation and an eclectic approach with cognitive + behaviorist + hypnotherapy)

B: Triple vaginal exercises and/or training, education with feedback

C: Factors related to the couple

Sub-Factors

a: Failed hypnosis treatment in the past

b: Existence of personality disorders and other mental illnesses

c: Blue-Eyed Girl Effect (Definition by Dr. Ulusoy)

d: Urine Incontinence Problem (Definition by Dr. Ulusoy)

e: Anatomical problems of the vagina or hymen

f: Fear of examination or inability to be examined, refusal of treatment

g: Erection problem – Seesaw Effect (Definition by Dr. Ulusoy)

h: The sexual trauma knowingly/unknowingly caused by the spouse. The man's behaviors that create sudden distrust.

i: One or both of the spouses not loving the other, sexual incompatibility or sexual repulsion disorder

j: Sexual frigidness

DR. ULUSOY METHOD IN VAGINISMUS TREATMENT – 1

Firstly, the method that I apply is given with its technical outlines, and then a new structuring is presented for therapist that will not be practicing examination or training.

The following Chapter 3 *Hypnosis and its Usage in Vaginismus* contains hypnosis suggestions to be used in the treatment formulations given here.

Do not forget! The vagina is loose in the Turkish woman! Something can go in through there. We are going to apply hypnotherapy on the contractions and uncontrollability of the body. Let the patient know this, too.

What is targeted with the patient?

1. Making her believe that she will succeed,
2. Giving her the courage to start,
3. Removing the contractions,
4. Confirming that something can go inside and that the diameter could increase, and whether there are any problems with the hymen,
5. Transferring of authority after the finger exercises and moving on to the penis stage,
6. Enabling breathing, leg spreading and hip control are the main objectives.

The Dr. Ulusoy Method utilizes **Psychoeducation + Cognitive Therapy + Behaviorist Therapy + Hypnotherapy** treatment methods. It is a treatment protocol that lasts for **three phases and one and a half days on average**. It is also referred to as *The Three-Stage Treatment Method/Technique*.

1. The patient's medical history is taken. (How long has she had it? Has she been to treatment before? Has she had a hymen operation? What reactions does she give during intercourse? Can she look or touch her genital region? Can she allow something into the vagina? What does hypnosis bring to her mind?)
2. Hypnosis pre-study is performed; the mechanism and details of what we going to do are explained. And an informed consent form is signed by the patient.
3. The patient's problem is formulated according to cognitive, behaviorist, dynamic and existentialist structures.

4. The subconscious and its working mechanism are explained with the psychoeducation.
5. The patient is mentally prepared for the therapy with The Dr. Ulusoy Hypnosis Induction Technique during the hypnosis pre-session.
6. The training film on vaginismus is watched by the woman and her partner.
7. A detailed psychoeducation on genital areas is provided for the patient and her partner.
8. Hypnotherapy, directed toward the problem formulated with the hypnotherapy session, is performed.
9. The patient is sent to the hotel to perform the first stage of the three-stage dildo homework.
10. Having completed the first homework, the patient is taken into hypnotherapy again and is sent to the hotel once again to perform the second homework.
11. After completing the second homework, the patient is taken into hypnotherapy again and she is sent to hotel one more time to do the homework that contains the exercises on transfer of finger authority and the training film about sex positions.
12. When the patient gives the information that the homework is done, she is called back the next morning. If there has been anything missing or anything she had not been able to do in the homework, a training with examination and exercises are performed to complete the homework during the day.
13. The next day, hypnotherapy is applied to the patient once again and she is sent to the hotel after being provided with a psychoeducation on how the intercourse will take place.
14. The treatment is over if the penis has entered completely. If only the head or half of it could enter, and if there are contractions, an additional hypnotherapy session is carried out and the remaining contractions are removed.
15. After success, ten-day dildo and intercourse exercises are prescribed to be done before and after menstruation for enhancement and compatibility.

The above fifteen articles are the guidelines of The Dr. Ulusoy Method. The patient arrives in the morning and we see her at intervals throughout the day to complete the therapies and exercises (Three phases). After seeing the patient the next day and carrying out another hypnotherapy session, they are sent to their hotel to have the experience. With an eclectic approach that targets the subconscious, results are obtained in an average of twenty-four to thirty-six hours (One and a half days).

DR. ULUSOY METHOD IN VAGINISMUS TREATMENT – 2

The Dr. Ulusoy Method-2, differently from Method-1, takes hypnosis as basis in vaginismus and it contains a 45-minute examination with feedback, and dilator exercises. It is a treatment that enables intercourse in the same day with a three-phase and three-hour work.

In this treatment, contractions are removed and the mind-body relaxation is provided with a formulated problem-oriented therapy comprising of a *Formulated Problem-Oriented approach + Mirror Neuroreactivation applied Psychoeducation + Hypnosis*. It is an eclectic, integrative and gradual treatment which is comprised of a process in which the model regarding the relationship is taught with a behaviorist education and treatment that includes *Preparation of the relationship model + Biofeedback + Mindfulness* as well as *Applied Holotropic Breathwork* for removal of resistances.

The treatment is directed toward learning and creating neuroplasticity in the brain/mind.

The reason why the treatment duration is so short is due to the fact that it works on the Psoas Muscle Group, which is the main factor in vaginismus, and I was the first one in the World to come up with this definition.

Other treatments work on the pelvic floor muscles with Kegel Exercises. Whereas in vaginismus, the vagina is loose and vaginismus has nothing to do with pelvic floor muscles. Therefore, other treatments last relatively longer.

As seen above, my treatment method follows a different path than other treatments and it has a dynamic structure.

In Method-2, the first eight steps of Method-1 are applied in the same way.

While the steps 9, 10 and 11 are given as homework at the hotel in Method-1, they are performed at our clinic in Method-2 with an examination including 45-minute feedback-assisted Holotropic Breathwork, Psoas control, relaxation and dilator exercises. When we are the ones who perform or make the patient perform such exercises, it makes learning easier and speeds up the process. After the examination and exercises, the patient is taken under hypnosis once again and suggestions on *Preparation for Intercourse* are given with *Hypnodrama and Ego Reinforcement*. Then she is given the training film on sex positions and sent to the hotel. At the hotel, she is asked to repeat the dilator exercise, which I had taught during examination and training. She watches the film on sex position afterwards. The patient is called back in the afternoon of the same day, and if there have been no problems in doing the homework, she is given ideomotor-assisted suggestions on intercourse under hypnosis, and they have intercourse in the evening.

The steps 12, 13, 14 and 15 are same as Method I. Only the 13th step is brought forward to the afternoon session of the same day. As seen, the time for treatment success between both methods may be reduced by twelve hours.

The question asked by our patients before they come is, "What is it doesn't happen?" to which we reply, "The treatment will end only when you say, 'We've done it!'"

Since it is directed toward learning, it will also be a permanent treatment. I stand by my treatment method at all times, rest assured.

THE FIVE-STEP GATE MODEL IN VAGINISMUS TREATMENT

"5-BK Model – Dr. Ulusoy, 2014" for psychologists and psychiatrists

Below, by using similar details as in the steps of The Dr. Ulusoy Method, the treatment is structured as finger homework over five steps rather than three, for psychologists and psychiatrists who will not be medically examining their patients or who will not be conducting exercises with them. The advised five steps may be planned daily, on every other day or on every week at most.

The Hanging Gardens of Babylon metaphor under the title *Hypnosis Usage in Vaginismus* in Chapter 3 could be used to emphasize the mind at the start of the 5-BK Model and at each step.

The Therapy Approach Structured for Psychologists and Psychiatrists

*This approach, which is the modified version of The Dr. Ulusoy Method for Vaginismus Treatment restructured for psychologists and psychiatrists, will hereaf-ter be called the **Five-Step Gate Model** or shortly, the **5-BK Model – Dr. Ulusoy.***

Make them use water-bases gels such as OK or Durex in their exercises. Tell them that you are thinking of reaching a solution in five sessions, if everything goes well. Passing from one step to the next depends on the practicability of the homework. If the homework is done, the gate opens and the other session will commence. If your patient has not done the homework or if she has left it halfway, it is evaluated as the gate not being open or the gate being half-open. And you should remain at the same step and work with hypnotherapy to provide the practicability of the homework. Make sure you point out the fact that the treatment process may not be a bed of roses but also that it is the permanence of the water that cuts through the marble, not the power.

I have written down the steps roughly for you to have some pre-cognition. You could spice them up with your intuitions and experiences.

If possible, make sure that the time between each session is no longer than a week. It could make your work easier if it is shorter.

Point out to her that there could be stinging, burning or tingling feelings during the exercises, and that it is normal. But also tell her that she should let you know if she feels a cutting, piercing pain, in which case you may continue the exercises with anesthetic pomades. The cutting, piercing pain indicates a problem at the hymen.

During finger exercises, she needs to inhale slowly through the nose and gradually move her finger, which she has placed at the vagina entrance, inwards as she exhales slowly from the mouth. She should continue inwards one stage (2-3 mm or 0.2-0.4 inches, it is best to leave it to the patient) with each exhaling. She is not allowed to take the finger back out during the exercise, she can wait at the same position, take a few deep breaths but then she needs to continue from the point she has stopped. The exercise must not be interrupted until the finger is completely inside. She can do the finger exercise by herself, or she can have her partner do it. They are free on that. When the vagina starts taking the finger inside, she will feel hotness, slipperiness and a gritty, velvet-like structure, let her know this in advance. At the first 0.8 to 1.2 inches of the entrance, she will feel the fleshy elevations, which I call lower and upper cushions, and after passing this point, she will be entering a larger area; tell her what she will be experiencing.

In fragile-built women, the finger and the upper wall of the vagina entrance may become stuck between the pelvic bone and cause pain; keep this in mind.

First Step, Gate 1

1. Formulize the problem. Let the patient see this with a quadruple formulation on paper or on the white board.
2. Point out that the main problem is the contractions in the body and that

you will be applying gradual hypnotherapy sessions for this. Tell her that you will be working with visualizations in the mind and other hypnotherapy techniques.

3. Provide an anatomic psychoeducation on the vagina, the uterus and their neighborhoods.
4. Make her do breathing exercises, using the diaphragm.
5. Conduct a pre-hypnosis session. Work on relaxation and carry out hypnosis preparations for the following steps. Leave metaphors in the mind.
6. Give them the vaginismus training DVD for her to watch with her partner before the next session.

Second Step, Gate 2

1. Ask for their comments on the video.
2. Tell her that she will be doing finger exercises. Provide psychoeducation primarily on leg separation, breathing control, finding the vagina entrance with her finger and directing the finger inside during the finger exercises.
3. Take her into hypnotherapy. Give her relaxation suggestions + Provide the same psychoeducation you had just given earlier under hypnosis this time (Lozanov) + Give courage and confidence suggestions + Ensure her that she will not any feel pain while working in that region, and that she can tolerate it even if she does feel any + Simulate the homework.
4. She needs to take one finger inside, one node at a time, at home. It is enough for her to do it four or five times.

Third Step, Gate 3

(If the homeworks of the second session could not be done; investigate the problem and use the hypnotherapy technique to remove the problem. If the homeworks are done, proceed.)
1. Give her two fingers and three nodes exercise and psychoeducation.
2. Provide relaxation with hypnotherapy + Give psychoeducation for two fingers exercise under hypnosis, and also make her simulate the homework + Support her ego. It is enough for her to do it four or five times.

Forth Step, Gate 4

(If the homeworks of the third session could not be done; investigate the problem and use the hypnotherapy technique to remove the problem. If the homeworks are done, proceed.)

1. Provide psychoeducation for three fingers and two nodes. This exercise should be done by twenty times by herself and then twenty times by her partner.
2. Start giving suggestions about the experience and intercourse with hypnotherapy. Make her simulate the homework and the experience.

Fifth Step, Gate 5

(If the homeworks were successful, you have come to the point of trial. If not, you will need to work on the problems with hypnotherapy)
1. Provide psychoeducation on what kind of experience they will have. Use pictures to explain the positions and the ways of approaching.
2. Give them the sex positions DVD and let them watch it at home.
3. Tell them to do the two and three finger exercises* before the experience, and to leave some gel inside. After placing the penis at the vagina entrance, they are to do the directing moves. They need to try at least two positions with her on top and below.
4. Repeat the psychoeducation in hypnotherapy. Work on relaxation and have her simulate the experience.

* During these exercises, dilators with at least three different lengths and diameters could also be used instead of fingers.

COMPARISON OF CLASSICAL TREATMENTS WITH THE DR. ULUSOY METHOD

Classical behaviorist treatments last for approximately twelve weeks. They are carried out with weekly meetings.
1. Getting to know the bodies in the first weeks
2. Forbidding of intercourse
3. Romance-oriented approaches
4. Week by week work, starting from one finger one node to two fingers three nodes
5. Having the same exercises done by the man
6. Passing to the penis phase

Due to the fact that classical treatments are long and require intensive exercises, the failure rate during treatment is increased.

1. Some cases are unable to do finger exercises
2. Some cases cannot continue long-term treatment
3. Some cases cannot succeed in the penis-vagina relationship after completing the finger exercises because the mind is not ready, meaning that the exercises have only been mechanical

Whereas The Dr. Ulusoy Method,

1. Does not involve intensive finger exercises. It utilizes finger exercises for very short terms and for the transfer of authority.
2. Does not forbid sex.
3. Focuses on the problem and emotions, and applies solutions specific for the individual.
4. Prepares the mind first with the cognitive, behaviorist approach and with the hypnotherapy methods developed specifically for vaginismus, thus rendering the three-phase exercises on the vagina doable within a short period of time.
5. Includes examination with feedback and Holotropic Breathwork for Psoas Muscle control and relaxation, as well as dilator exercises.
6. Enables the patient, who has arrived in the morning, to be ready for the penis/intercourse in the evening after a total work of three hours.

Due to the facts that it doesn't last long, that it comprises easy exercises and that it goes on with learning, it is also efficient in patients who have applied to many places without success. It is a treatment directed toward learning, and behind the scenes of learning in such short period is the highly effective hypnotherapy.

SUCCESS STORIES WITH THE DR. ULUSOY METHOD

Sample Case

Hello,

March 22 has been the turning point of my life. I got rid of the vaginismus that I thought to be unbeatable. I am happy, peaceful and I can look around with a smile now. Thanks to Dr. Murat Ulusoy. Even at times when I thought I couldn't do it, you gave me the confidence that I had it in me to succeed. Thanks for everything. Classical treatment, botox, anesthetic pomades, alcohol, muscle relaxant drugs are all factors that cause waste of time for vaginismus. I tried them all. And you also become mentally depressed as time passes by. You need to be treated immediately, without losing much time. There wasn't a single doubt while going to Kuşadası Town because, above all, I had complete faith in my doctor. Owing to Dr. Murat Ulusoy (His mastery + reassurance + positive approach) we managed it in one and a half days. If I did it, so can you.

Best regards,

Sample Case

Hi ☺

Hello again, Mr. Murat. ☺ I guess I'll be sending you thank you e-mails whenever I think about it. I had come to you in February. You solved my 1.5-year problem in 1.5 days. In a short time, I became able to have a pleasureful intercourse. As if I had never dealt with such a problem. When you realize that it was doable, you get angry with yourself for waiting 1.5 years. I not only got rid of vaginismus owing to you, but I also regained my self-confidence. I thank you once again for the interest and consideration you have displayed toward my husband and me. You already gave us your blessing but I want to talk about it on every occasion. Please let your other patients read my e-mail. Please don't let them lose time. Apparently it was not an incurable illness; and the correct address is you, of course. They should come to you before getting worn out, both financially and mentally, and before losing time. Right now, I feel as if I have never had vaginismus. I hope my e-mails will be helpful to other women who are in the same situation that I was. I also had worries before coming to you, but when I saw you and talked to you, I said, "Good thing I came here." I had told my husband especially that I trusted Mr. Murat and that we should go. My trust has not come to naught; I thank you for this too. Right now, we are enjoying our marriage but if we ever think of having children, I am planning on naming him/her *Ada* as in Kuşadası. ☺ You are a perfect person both professionally and personally; what else can I say…

Sample Case
Hello, Mr. Murat.

I want to share my joy and happiness of my five-week pregnancy with you and with the members of the group.

As you will also remember, we had applied to you for treatment from France in 2010. Those days that I thought would never pass are long gone. Now we are living the excitement of having a child. I can't help but recall how experienced, quick and confidant you were in this field every time I come across web sites of doctors who cure vaginismus in treatments lasting weeks or months. As long as you are here, vaginismus is not a difficult illness at all. It is a condition that quickly goes away in one and a half days. I advise vaginismus patients not to exaggerate such a simple illness. With doctors like you, of course… God bless you.

Sample Case
Good morning, Mr. Murat.

Could you please share the e-mail below with the group?

By the way, whenever you look at the pigeon I gave you, please remember my gratitude and thanks for helping me get rid of this situation. We had the joy of solving it in one and a half days.

Thanks again for everything; I hope to meet you with more happy news. Take very good care of yourself. ☺

Endless thanks for rendering the depths of my mind as free as the free pigeon of Kuşadası. With love…

Sample Case
Hello my dear group friends.

Those who have been following may remember; I had written in July that I had an appointment with Mr. Murat and that I was counting the days until the time I would share with you the happiness of succeeding, as did all the other friends who have managed it…

I, who had been reading every success message from the group with tears and who had been thinking whether I could be able to beat this thing that never left my mind and gnawed at my brain for two years, am now writing this e-mail with tears of joy. ☺ I managed it too, in one and a half days!

I went to Mr. Murat in the morning with trembling hands… His sincere attitude and good humor starts from the moment he opens the door, and you start treatment after the open and clear answers to everything on your mind, even before you ask them. And even you cannot believe what you have been able to achieve in such short time. Leave your hesitations, question marks and all your doubts behind because I used to have them too, but they are gone away now. If you really want to solve this problem, go to Mr. Murat without confusing yourself, without wearing yourself out and without spending money on places where you won't be cured, and you will be rid of this psychological state in a short time. I have just come back from a dreamlike vacation last weekend (Actually I called it the real honeymoon ☺). And I left all my question marks and fears into the deep blue sea and skies of Kuşadası, thanks to Mr. Murat. I feel like I've remarried my husband. I can now look into my husband's eyes with a smile and when I hold his hands tight, I just remember his support for all this time in getting rid of this problem. And every time I think of that, I fall in love with him once again and feel grateful for having him in my life. If your husband has also supported you and waited patiently until the end of this problem, I say that you should think that he, before you, has the right to enjoy this happiness, and motivate yourself this way as you start your treatment. That was what I did from the first step and we overcame this problem with the support of my husband… What happens after treatment? All there is left for you to do is to enjoy the beautiful and happy moments that await you after achieving the comfort of having lifted the world's weight off your shoulders, and you become able to approach other people smilingly because there are no more question marks left in your head… In order to experience all this, first you need to go to Mr. Murat without wasting any time. ☺ The rest is up to you. ☺
Love…

Sample Case
Hello, Mr. Murat.

We had made an appointment with you in July 2011 and we had gotten rid of this illness very quickly. Of course it was not that easy. While waiting for four years, I suffered both financially and also mentally with my efforts to persuade my husband, as we both coped with hopelessness. Thankfully, first with the grace of God and then with your efforts, I have finally gotten rid of this problem. May God help everyone in this situation to heal. I too, was very hesitant before coming to you. But it was not because of you. I was having doubts because of my lack of self-confidence and because of the psychological pressure my husband had inflicted. Because if I hadn't been healed again, there would be no place for the word *treatment* in our lives.

Please trust the Doctor. If you have the means, please don't spend time anywhere else. Don't waste your money. Even though I had very difficult times, I waited patiently. Dear Mr. Murat was our first and only doctor. Instead of the months-long disappointment, get rid of this burden in a period of 1.5 – 2 days.

I thank you very much, and wish you health and welfare so you can successfully make other patients smile, like me. I hope everything goes your way, Doctor. I will be following your group, your e-mails. I hope I'll get back to you with even better news.

Sample Case
Hello.

My husband and I had gone to Mr. Murat in November 2011 for the treatment we wanted so badly. Indeed, we smoothly went through all the phases of the treatment in 1.5 days, thanks to the Doctor, and we returned home from Kuşadası with a peaceful mind, in the psychology of returning from a vacation. Thankfully, we feel as if we have never had this problem that we hadn't been able to overcome during the six years of our marriage. Now we are able to experience it comfortably and moreover, we are getting better at it every day. Actually I used to have an extreme aversion due to failing for six years. This problem went away slowly, and even further, the pain and fear have gone away completely. You really cannot believe yourself. I mean, not being able to do it for so many years while it was so easy... My only regret is; why did we wait for six years? Actually I was only able to find Mr. Murat through his web site after five years. Those of you who are having this problem; don't worry yourself and reach Mr. Murat as soon as possible. The rest is easy. I prayed God so much to be rid of this problem and He sent Mr. Murat as his instrument. Thank God.

Thank you very much, Doctor. I was wondering if I would be able to write a success e-mail and now my dream has come true. I will always keep following your web site. I recommend you to everyone.

Sample Case
Hello.

We were at Kuşadası in May for treatment. We returned after leaving behind the biggest burden of my life, which I had carried for the first six months of our marriage. It has been two years after it and we feel as if we have never lived those days. While writing you this e-mail, I am also looking at my daughter sleeping on my lap. She is one-year-old now. I am a bit obsessed with keeping things from days that I deem important. And the month of May is very special for me; both because it was the time I was treated and also because we had had our missing honeymoon… The bus tickets for the trip to Kuşadası, the brochures of the hotel we stayed at, the business card of the cabstand that took us from the bus station…I've kept them all. Now I look at them with a smile.☺ Beautiful memories from the last day of the bad times. ☺ My husband was my greatest supporter before the treatment, and my greatest fear was to lose him one day because of the problems this illness would cause…

Please don't make wrong choices that will ruin your life. I did not exhaust myself anywhere else and went to Mr. Murat. Thanks to Mr. Murat's support, I now have a more solid, happy home and a daughter. And I wouldn't change any of these for the World…

Sample Case
Hello, my friends.

I tried to continue my marriage while suffering from the same problem for five years. In 2011, I went to Mr. Murat for treatment and got rid of my problem in a period of one and a half days. In the first year of my marriage, I reached Mr. Murat on the internet and waited with great patience. I didn't apply to any other place for treatment. I didn't have money to spend around. Please take your husband and go directly to Mr. Murat and let your life change in a day. Let your silent cries end. As one of his patients, I thank Mr. Murat very much. I pray to God that I will be able to give the news of my baby one day. May God help you get rid of your problems. He had made our hearts and eyes smile. Goodbye…

Sample Case
October 2012, a story of success…

Easy to say, five whole years…

We still don't know what dragged us to Kuşadası with great motivation after our long research and after leaving behind long and stressful five whole years. In October 2012, before the Sun came out, we set out on the Dr. Ulusoy path and we returned, leaving behind our illness that was solved in only 1.5 days. We were already whole emotionally but there were mountains and walls between us in the physical sense. We returned that day, leaving in that hotel room all those distressful, unhappy days when I thought I was abusing my husband's compassion and love, when I read my doctor's e-mails in tears, when I thought whether I would be able to share my success story one day, when I was dying to have a baby and when I had become selfish, unable to be happy with pregnancy news, when I woke up crying, most importantly, when I wasn't able to feel my womanhood, and when I just couldn't pass to womanhood even though I had given up on my teenage years long ago. Now we are truly man and wife in our home. If you are sitting at your computer right now and reading these lines in tears, then you are the one that I am trying to reach out to. Never ever think that I was privileged, that I was in better condition than you are, and that was why I healed. We all have the same problem. So immediately go to Dr. Ulusoy, as I did without taking any wrong routes, without trying any other physician. He will meet you at the door with his wonderful timbre, saying your name and last name. You will meet someone who will not let you deal with anyone else and who will fight with you -more than you will- until your problem goes away. And probably, he will not remain someone that you see once in your life and leave. Believe me; the first thought you will have after the first treatment will be waiting for the day that you will visit him with your baby. You will never ever believe what you were able to achieve with him. Just as you are unsuccessful right now, you will be so much successful while being treated by him. You don't know how you do it, but you do it. My greatest reservation was hypnosis. You can't believe how much I'm laughing at myself right now. You just sit there with your eyes closed. The only difference in that your doctor is loading you with wonderful messages with his wonderful tone. I could go under hypnosis right now; that is how much I liked listening to beautiful stories. ☺ After the hypnosis, some people were talking about homework on their e-mails, and I was very scared of the homework, thinking, "Oh God, what if I can't do the homework..." He told me and I did them, watching myself in disbelief. My husband and I completed our homework in amazement, like two hardworking students. ☺ So the take-home message is; our conscious can deceive us, but no problem, because there is also Dr. Ulusoy who can tame the conscious.☺ So, what I'm trying to say is; believe in yourself and your strength with the right doctor and the right treatment. If a coward like me could succeed, all of you can, too. Don't wait, go, go and feel your womanhood.

As for you Doctor, neither my husband nor I could find the words to express our gratitude. I hope we will meet somewhere again, the four of us. ☺ We will have flowers in our hands again, and you will have love on your face... We owe you a great debt of gratitude. You can be assured that, in our hearts, we will be carrying the Dr. Ulusoy name, which we have engraved in our lives, with thanks and indebtedness.

With regards and love…

Remain with the light…

INFORMED CONSENT FORM

You have applied to us with vaginismus (Inability to have intercourse) problem. During our treatment process, your anamnesis (The history of your illness) will be taken, the reasons of your illness will be determined with the quadruple (Cognitive, behaviorist, dynamic, existentialist) formulation and you will be taught, with The Dr. Ulusoy Hypnosis Model, how to relax and control your breathing, your mind and body. Hypnosis is an intermittent stage between sleep and wakefulness. Your conscious will be kept open during the treatment process, and the faulty learning processes of your subconscious will be replaced with new ones. There will be no retrogression during hypnosis to obtain information; with analytical hypnotherapy (Due to the principle of the mind creating fantasies and distorting reality) you will be aware of everything at all times and you will learn step-by-step how to relax and control your mind and body. In our treatment process, hypnosis will be used as a technique to speed up learning and to replace contractions with relaxation. Your problem will be formulated, and suggestions directed to that problem and that feeling will be provided. As we will be working in a problem-oriented manner, suggestions that you do not want, or suggestions that could disrupt your personality integrity will not be given. The Dr. Ulusoy Hypnosis Model that will be applied is a process focused on the mind-body relaxation so there are no risks or complications.

Concerning your problem, you will be provided with verbal/visual or, if necessary, one-on-one training accompanied by practice/examination, where you will be learning about your genital structures.

The history taking of your illness, the formulation and hypnotherapy will be done with you one-on-one in the session room, while your partner is able to watch you on our closed circuit system, without sound. Only our therapy sessions are being video recorded. As per ethical rules, such recordings are not published anywhere.

After being organized in a way that your identity information will not be exposed, your success story may be published in written form on our web site, in printed media or in the contents of a book.

If your physician sees the need to perform the exercises about your learning and application process regarding your genital area, your partner will be with you and support you.

During your treatment process, there may be other therapy options that your physician deems necessary for the healing of your illness, and examinations directed toward training, and perhaps medical drug use in case of necessity.

At the vaginal region, triple (Rarely quadruple, if found necessary) short, easy vaginal exercises with feedback will be conducted. After your mind is prepared, we will first wait for you to be able to perform them by yourself (85% of our cases that were unable to allow anything inside were able to do this easily after the mind is prepared). In cases when they cannot be performed due to an incapableness related to personality structure or due to lack of courage, the exercises will be performed by your physician accompanied by examination and training.

During the vaginal exercises, your hymen may become deformed and you may lose your virginity. Although four out of ten hymens are elastic and allow penetration without bleeding, there could be partial bleeding from the deformed hymen area. If problems are anticipated at your hymen, the exercises will be done painlessly by local use of medicine. Rarely, there could be superficial irritations, rashes, infections, vaginal injuries and bleedings due to the work done on the vagina entrance and inside. If such complications occur, the necessary medical precautions will be taken by your physician.

If you do not receive treatment, it is a very small probability that your illness will heal on its own. Sexuality is a strong bond that is able to provide family unity among couples and that can solve the craving for motherhood. In couples that do not get treated, the love and respect of the couple toward each other may diminish in time, and it may turn into a stressful process that could lead to divorce.

As per ethical rules and due to the fact that we are working on human beings, 100% treatment success cannot be guaranteed. Statistically, the majority of our patients, who apply and who complete the treatment process, are able to solve their problem permanently in a short time. With our knowledge, competence and experience, we will work to do our best to solve your problem under the best circumstances. Even if there is a failure, we will make sure that you will not suffer financially.

In vaginismus treatment, the harmony between the patient, her partner and the physician is essential. Just like a trivet, all three legs must be on solid ground. We have to maintain this harmony during your treatment process.

You will be followed up by your physician before, during and after your treatment.

If you unilaterally decide to stop, discontinue treatment after it starts, not only will your problem remain unsolved but it could also go into a more difficult period.

After your consent is received and after payment is done, if you unilaterally decide to stop, abandon treatment after it starts, there will be no refunding due to the fact that we are working on a schedule and because we dedicate an intensified period of one and a half day to three days for each patient.

Once you start treatment and give your consent, you are required to remain in the treatment process until your treatment is ended by your physician.

Our treatment duration with The Dr. Ulusoy Method is one and a half days on average. If there are any problems related to your personality, physical structures or erectile dysfunctions, it could extend up to three days. After your treatment is over and after you have had the experience, you will be given extra exercises for before and after menstruation in order to reinforce your education.

During the treatment, we rarely come across *personality disorders* or *blue-eyed girl effect*, in which case the treatment may be extended. If the time you have allocated for the treatment proves insufficient or if we need to give you extra exercises for longer terms, your treatment follow-up will be done online.

A pleasureful sexuality starts with fantasies and dreams in the mind. During your treatment, you will be informed on this matter with suggestions and at the end of your treatment, you will be supported with necessary training tools. As for the pleasure, you will need to enter a new learning period in your life.

Once you are treated and have intercourse, your illness will not repeat itself in terms of the problems we have dealt with. If there is any reoccurrence of the problem due to these reasons, your treatment will also be repeated without any additional cost.

Other than this, in the years following your treatment, a secondary vaginismus could develop due to contractions and closure of the lower vagina muscles because of a psychologic trauma with the partner and an existentialist effect, or after a problematic or stressful normal delivery where the physician or the midwife applies force, or due to molestation or rape. In such case, the formation mechanism (Ethiology) of the vaginismus is different so a separate therapy application could be required.

Dr. Murat Ulusoy

I have read what my physician has written about the treatment of my illness, the treatment process, complications and post treatment. I have listened to him and received satisfactory answers to my questions. My partner/spouse and I accept the medical applications and the treatment process, which my physician, Dr. Murat Ulusoy, has advised and which he will advise later during the treatment process for the solution of my vaginismus problem.

Date:

Patient _____   Partner/Spouse _____

Name and Last Name: Name and Last Name:

Signature: Signature:

ID number: ID number:

Address:

CHAPTER 3

HYPNOSIS AND ITS USE IN VAGINISMUS

In this chapter, you will reach information on hypnosis inductions, deepening techniques and how they are used in vaginismus, as well as information prepared specifically for this purpose. This chapter is designed for therapists.

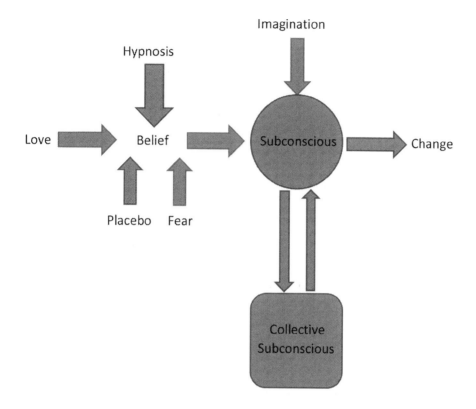

This drawing emphasizes the fact that hypnosis, love/compassion, placebo and fear can affect the subconscious via belief and also that they can initiate change. Whereas hypnotic imaginations and -as the Sufis[4] say- creative prayers/ images reach the subconscious directly. One needs to think of change in the broad sense, as the realization of spiritual, mental, emotional, somatic/physical, and biotic dreams. At the same time, the subconscious also reaches the collective subconscious, defined by Jung. Synchronicity and coincidences also belong to the collective. As Shams once said, "Everyone is connected to each other with invisible strings."

---

(4)   **TN:** Sufis are those who practice Sufism (Also known as Tasawwuf), variously defined as "Islamic mysticism", characterized by particular values, ritual practices, doctrines and institutions, and represents "the main manifestation and the most important and central crystallization of" mystical practice in Islam.

HYPNOSIS, BELIEF AND CHANGE

Ever since mankind has existed, he has had the inclination toward believing in something. Even atheists have a belief system to support their lives.

While looking for the answer to the question, "What is the thing that causes psychological and psychosomatic illness?" I thought there could be a key. It had to be such a key that it should, on its own or as a catalyst, be able to provide speedy healing when added to thoughts or therapies. Was there really such a thing? Or was I dreaming of castles in the sky? Was there something else, smiling to us sweetly behind the activity we simply called placebo?

Yes, the key I am talking about is *BELIEF*! You exist if you believe. It is not so important want you believe in. Right or wrong, it is important that you believe something. In illnesses, if you cannot get any response despite all the therapies you have applied, it is because you are not convincing. To put a finer point on it, if the person is conditioned to produce negative thoughts and if she unknowingly believes in them, you cannot overcome such a belief with a lower or same degree belief. You can provide healing only if you can replace the patient's belief system, which she has created for her existence, with a higher belief.

As one of my consultees once wrote to me: "I want to consult you about my mother. She constantly lives in the past and in negativity. She keeps on remembering the bad things form her past. Of course she also remembers the positive things but at a very low rate."

Her positive thought just cannot have any effect because of her acceptance and belief in the past and the negativities. Perhaps someway, knowingly or not, the subconscious is doing this in order to realize herself in her environment.

Why was Erickson successful? He had an agile mind based on observation.

How was Mesmer able to provide healing in his time?

It is possible to give more examples. What lies beneath are charisma and plausibility...

The actual questions we have to ask ourselves are,
1. Through which mechanism does belief influence the body?
2. How can we create belief and use it in the healing of illnesses?

The existing therapy approaches are directed toward the mind and its mental functions, and related to organizing the structure of the body and the conscious. But the belief of being sick or healthy can also have effects on the body and the mind. The ability to activate belief is the nourishment of the soul, the kindling of the spirit's fire.

When we touch the hands of subjects, who are under deep trance with hypnosis, with a piece of iron and tell them that it is red-hot, or in other words, when we convince the system, we see that erythema (Redness) and bulla (Blister) are formed on the skin as if touched by hot fire.

When you do the same thing while the subject is not under hypnosis, you cannot get the same result. So, this situation can occur in the *altered state of consciousness* that has the highest potential of cogency. In other words, it occurs in situations when the discernment of the conscious is removed or when the conscious is directed toward another area.

So, in therapies, we have to create an altered situation at the conscious. Afterwards, we can also apply several other therapy approaches under hypnosis.

Therefore, we need to give key suggestions or patterns after altering the conscious, and this can be done by activating the belief schemes. Wrong information, defined as *faulty learning*, could better be defined as *Faulty Learning Belief.*

We may learn a wrong piece of information but not every wrongly learnt information causes problems for us. What create the problem are *thoughts or engrams loaded with emotions.* But emotions on their own also don't seem to be effective. Sometimes during hypnosis sessions, emotional discharges are experienced, partial healing is provided but this is not effective on its own. While the accumulated emotions are discharged during hypnosis, at the same time, we need to reshape learning with cognitive and behaviorist therapy approaches.

I would like to give you a few examples from my own life. While walking around in the neighborhood bazaar with my son (Five or six years old), suddenly I lost sight of him. At that moment, dozens of emotions passed through my mind in the form of snapshots, all of them negative. Everything from him being kidnapped by the organ mafia to him being kidnapped by people who wanted to do me harm… When I gathered myself, I looked around in great haste. I called the police. Then I thought of calling his mother's workplace. With the fear he felt when he could not see me, he had run to his mother's office which was about a mile away. Afterwards, I began developing symptoms of panic every time I walked in crowded places. I was holding his hand very tightly and I was in distress all the time. It felt as if he would get lost any minute. My son started having similar complaints, too. He was too worried to leave my side. I began encouraging him and I led him to increase his belief factors, to feel confidence. I was saying that he could do it and I would wait a few steps behind as I waited for him to finish the job at hand. He used to turn and look behind in great worry. With each thing he managed to do, I fueled his belief in success and self-confidence. This way, I had been able to replace the lack of confidence my son was displaying, with a greater belief and behavior model.

How can we develop the belief that can cope with all the problems? You always need to have a plan B; no matter how much distress you are in, your belief should be able to give you a new hope of life. You need to have not one but more goals in life.

If we show belief as a vector that extends left and right from point zero, the left side will consist of negative beliefs resulting from sorrow or distress, and the right side will be showing the positive beliefs, happy emotions and euphoric structure. Around point zero are our automated thoughts and our monotonous life style. If we cannot take our beliefs in the negative direction under control, they will create damage in our body just as the cancer cases triggered by extreme sorrow, major depressions or panic attacks; we will get into a vicious cycle like the mythological snake that bites its own tail. We try to get out of this vicious cycle by creating changes in our emotions, behaviors and thoughts with therapy support.

In life, negative beliefs don't always create negativity; sometimes it could be useful to utilize them. For instance, during the Battle of Gallipoli, Seyit Ali had transformed a negative environment into physical strength with the thoughts and belief of saving his country that was under enemy attack. He had lifted a 600 lb. ball and placed it into the cannon in one scoop.

On the other hand, positive beliefs could create bodily responses strong enough to beat cancer. Positive beliefs help you directly in leaping to your target point, while negative beliefs -if transformed- will indirectly help you do so.

For instance, I could have written this book with two kinds of motivations.
1. I could have written it with the belief that I will be very happy and useful when I put the book at the disposal of mankind (Positive belief).
2. I could have written it to create a new target or sustenance point for myself after an emotional breakdown I have gone through (Indirect use of negative belief).

As seen above, we can use either positive or negative belief systems to initiate a situation. The first one uses the positive belief system and the second one uses the negative belief system.

So, for a healthy mind and body, we need to have positive belief systems and we also need to turn on the inner generator that can transform our negative belief systems for indirect use.

And this is exactly where hypnosis applications come in handy. They activate the *Intelligent Mind* inside us. As Erickson said, "It is the subconscious that creates and also solves the problem." While the techniques applied in hypnosis enable us to activate our inner resources that solve the problem, they also aim to free the subconscious potentials from the limitations of the conscious.

The conclusion to be drawn is that an inner stimulus is required to direct the negative beliefs toward the target, such as in our proverb, "No Godsend arrives unless the subject is backed into a corner." If we are not able to provide this stimulus, mental disorders are formed as result of the vicus circle.

A paranoid thought could come to anyone's mind, such as, "Is my spouse cheating on me?" If you don't believe in this thought, it cannot be evaluated as a paranoid disorder.

What enhances belief?
1. Frequent repetitions
2. Increasing of probabilities
3. Fear and anxiety
4. Forbearance

In short, it is my opinion that in the hypnosis mechanism of action *lies the inactivation of the conscious control and the convincing of the subconscious, or the replacing of old beliefs that create the illness with new and healthy beliefs.*

NEGATIVE THOUGHTS (BELIEFS) ARE THE BASES OF ALL ILLNESSES!

I have always read and researched the philosopher physicians of the past with great envy. Although they did not have any microscopes or sufficient medicine, they were able to provide solutions with good observations and a creative mind. Of course, such solutions did not appear in their minds out of nowhere; the fact that they had a lot of knowledge on various topics enabled them to view events from a wider perspective. For instance, when you look at the life of Ibn Sina[5], you will see that he was interested in many topics such as philosophy, astronomy, medicine and religion.

As a matter of fact, although he had not given it a name, he was the one who came up with the concept of subconscious, when he said, "A spiritual imagination exists. The body has to obey the orders of this imagination. Not only can this imagination heal illnesses, it can also create illnesses out of nothing..."

The visualization studies done abroad in the last fifty years are in support of this. So, any positive structure we can create in thoughts (Willpower – Conscious - Left Brain) or in visualizations (Subconscious - Right Brain) will support us. But how much are we aware of this? Or are we driving our vehicle without fully knowing our system? Yes, unfortunately many people don't know themselves even if they arrive at a certain age, and neither do they try. Who are we, why are we on this Earth, if animals and humans are naturally able to experience the altered conscious state, why was this given to us by the Creator? Are we aware of what we are capable of doing with our minds and bodies?

One part of the answer to this multi-question riddle in terms of knowing ourselves, is positive our thoughts, or thought systems. When we open our eyes to this World, we are equipped with a physical organic hardware and a collective subconscious as Jung has declared; and we also have instinctual behaviors and reflexes. Apart from these, we use our five senses to load the software that will make it easier for our hardware to operate, and we constantly add new data.

If you were a computer programmer, would you write a program by assuming that it would create problems on the computers it is used, or assuming that it would not work? No, right? Then why on earth do we keep on writing

---

(5)   **TN:** Ibn Sina, often known in the West as Avicenna, was a Persian polymath who is regarded as one of the most significant physicians, astronomers, thinkers and writers of the Islamic Golden Age, and the father of early modern medicine.

faulty lines while programming ourselves? And why can't we correct these faulty lines by ourselves?

There is only one meaningful reason for this, the fact that we don't think we can change ourselves… The fact that we don't believe that we can heal ourselves… Perhaps because we have not been guided that way. Illnesses suddenly appear in us with unknown reasons and we trust physicians, psychologists, medicine for their treatment. Sometimes we cannot do without these. But if you don't supply the wish and will to be healed, and if you don't feel confident in the treatment inside, you will face a problematic healing period. Especially if you don't look for the responsibility for the illness within yourself and if you don't want to take this responsibility during the healing process, you will see that you are not healing, and then you will take it a step further, going door-to-door seeking help from clergymen or psychics.

Again, Ibn Sina says, "There is no incurable illness. There are patients who don't have the intention to be cured."

The important thing is to seek the cure inside yourself. And this is possible with positive beliefs and imagination…

"The mind does what it imagines and believes. The rest are details for the mind…" Dr. Ulusoy.

WHAT IS CLINICAL HYPNOSIS?

The meaning of the word hypnosis is *an intermittent stage between sleep and wakefulness*. It describes a state where there is mental and physical relaxation, where suggestibility is increased. It could be divided into three phases as light, intermediate and deep trance.

The important thing in hypnosis is not the depth but to manage change in the mind with the applied techniques. Hypnosis may be used by related people after a certain training. Hypnosis is a tool; the important thing is for this tool to be used correctly. In short, techniques that can provide change under hypnosis and that can cure the illness are required. I define hypnosis applications with these techniques as *Clinical Hypnosis*.

Let's imagine an iceberg. Let the horizontal yellow arrow, the part that is above water, represent the conscious, and let the part under water be the subconscious. Therapies, other than hypnosis, may come across negative emotions/resistance and remain deficient in reaching the subconscious and managing change. Whereas the problem-oriented techniques and suggestions in hypnosis can by-pass the resistance and directly influence the subconscious. Every suggestion given to the subconscious is like a seed planted in thought. It will bush out and start to grow either immediately or after a short while.

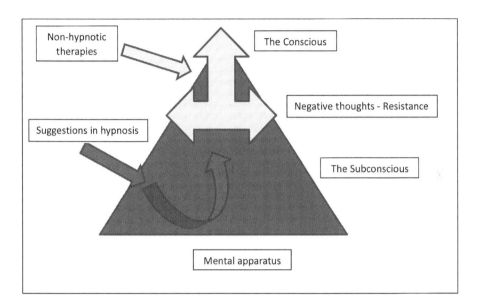

HYPNOSIS USAGE IN GYNECOLOGICAL DISEASES, WOMEN'S SEXUALITY AND CHILDBIRTH

1. Fear of coitus
2. Psychosexual problems
3. Menopause complaints
4. Dysmenorrhea (Painful menstruation)
5. Vaginismus
6. Deficient orgasm (Clitoral or vaginal) or lack thereof
7. Frigidity (Lack of sexual desire)
8. Dyspareunia (Painful sexual intercourse)

9. Nymphomania (Extreme desire for sex)
10. Fear of pregnancy
11. Nausea and vomiting of pregnancy
12. Fear of miscarriage
13. Painless delivery

HYPNOSIS INDUCTION TECHNIQUES

Induction is sine qua non in this business. Actually it could be called 50% of it. The prerequisite for treatment is for you to create a good induction in your patient. (Induction is valid for classical hypnosis. In Ericksonian Hypnosis, the subconscious is changed by using its own working mechanisms.) There are many induction techniques. As a matter of fact, it is said that there are as many induction techniques as there are therapists in the World. Your toolbox needs to be rich with induction techniques because it is only possible to reach resistant patients with different techniques. It is suggested that you participate in trainings and learn induction practically. In this book, *The Dr. Ulusoy Hypnosis Induction Technique* will be explained in detail. In addition, other induction techniques will also be mentioned for your practical use.

Some hypnosis induction techniques are actually aptitude tests.

Falling Back

The subject is standing and looking across at the point of junction where the wall and the ceiling meet. We stand behind the subject. With our palms, we provide a reassuring touch at the subject's scapula.

"I want you to focus all your attention on the point I have told you. Now take three deep breaths and exhale slowly… At the end of the third breath, I want you to close your eyes voluntarily. One… Two… Three… Very good, now you can close your eyelids. I am right behind you, continuing to support your shoulders and back with my hands… Shortly, while I remove my hands from you, you will experience my hands pulling your body backwards like a magnet does to pins… As my hands move away from you… Your body is coming backwards…"

In this technique, we can stand next to the subject during the initial breathings and follow her breathing rhythm with our hand. After her eyelids are closed, we can get behind her, support her back with our palms and continue suggestions.

If the subject is very susceptible, she can fall back suddenly; the therapist needs to be careful with this.

Looking Up Test

The subject is sitting in an armchair. The subject is asked to look at her eyebrows without tilting her head back. While the subject is looking at her eyebrows, the suggestion is given, "*Your eyelids are getting heavy and closing… They continue to drop down… As they close completely, your eyelids are stuck to each other…*"

Braid's Application

The subject is in the armchair again. We hold the bright object in our hand above her eye level at a 45-degree angle. We talk to the subject, "*Now I want you to give all your attention to the bright object in my hand. All your attention is on the object… Your eyelids are getting heavier and they are closing…*" (We slowly lower our hand and the object it is holding. The subject's eyes and eyelids are following the object.) When the object reaches the subject's eye level, you will observe her eyelids closing.

The Subject Following Her Own Thumb with the Eye Fixation Technique

The subject is in a sitting position. She lifts her right hand and arm forward, up to head level. Her thumb is open and facing upward, other four fingers are in a fist. She is asked to focus all her attention on the nail of her thumb.

"*Now I want you to focus all your attention on your fingernail. Yes, that's good… While your arm slowly comes down, your eyelids will close together with your hand… When your arm has fallen down completely, your eyelids will become closed and you will fall into a deep sleep…*"

While the subject follows her thumb and arm, her eyelids become heavy and they are closed.

Hypnotizing with Visualization

Our subject is in the armchair; we are talking to her. "*Shortly, I will be taking you under hypnosis with your will. I want you to visualize your past good memories like a movie strip. Where would you be happy; at the seaside, walking in the forest, swinging in a hammock, lying in a prairie?"*

"Swinging in a hammock," says the subject.

"Okay, now I want you to close your eyes. Imagine that you are lying in a hammock... You are swaying slowly... As you sway, you feel the sweet spring breeze on your face... You can actually feel the smell of the spring flowers around you... You can even hear the happy laughters of the children playing on the grass a bit further... You have a tiredness from the spring season... As you sway, the things you feel around you with your senses feel like a lullaby... Now I will count from one to ten and you will enter a deep sleep in that hammock. One... Two... Three... You are sleeeeeeping... Four... Five... Six... You are sleeeeeeping deeeeeeper... Seven... Eight... Nine and ten... Deeeeeply... You are sleeeeeeping deeeeeply..."

Finger Locking Test

Our subject is sitting in the armchair; her eyes are open. We ask her to interlock her hand and fingers, and to keep them in front of herself.

"Now your fingers are locked into each other. From now on, I will start giving you suggestions. With the suggestion I am about to give you, your fingers will become interlocked and stuck together. Even if you try to free them, they will lock even tighter. Now inhale deeply and let it out slowly. Right now, your fingers are completely locking into each other and sticking. The locking becomes more and more strong. You cannot free them even if you try... Yes, try to separate them now... You can't free them, can you? Your hands are completely interlocked right now... I have control of your fingers... And right now, your eyelids are becoming heavier... They are closing... You are going into a deeeeep sleeeeeep..."

Arm Dropping Test

Our subject is sitting in the armchair. We take our subject's left or right arm into our palm, grasping it from the elbow, and hold it up.

"Now I want you to put all the weight of your arm onto my hand. Leave it all to me... Let me feel it in my hand like a paralyzed arm..."

When we feel that the subject has left her arm completely to our hand, we go on.

"Shortly, I will remove the support I am giving to your arm. When I draw my hand away, your arm will fall down onto the armchair and to your side. At the moment your arm falls, your eyelids will become heavy and close. And you

will have entered a deep sleep... One... Your eyelids are getting heavier... Two... Your arm is getting heavier... Three..."

We suddenly remove the support from her arm. As her arm falls down freely, the subject's eyelids also become heavy and close.

Hypnotizing with the Vanishing Dot and Color Hallucination

The subject is sitting in the armchair. A dot, at the size of a chickpea, is drawn in the middle of a blank letter paper stuck on the wall across the subject (Wall distance is 10-15 feet).

"*First you need to take a deep breath and exhale. Good... Now I want you to give all your attention to the dot. Don't ever close your eyes... (As a paradox, this is the suggestion that her eyes will close.) Yes, I want you to follow this dot. Shortly, you will see that the dot is slowly shaking... It will start shaking at its place... Yes, do you see it?*"

"Yes."

"*Now continue following it. The dot's vibrations are growing... It is making small circular movements... Can you see?*"

"Yes."

"*The small circular movements are growing... It is moving right and left, and up and down... Can you see?*"

"Yes."

"*And now the dot is becoming indistinct... You will become unable to see the dot... The dot is disappearing... The dot is gone... Can you see the dot?*"

"The dot is gone! I can't see the dot. Where's the dot?"

"*The dot has vanished... Now you just see the paper... Right?*"

"Yes."

"*Now I want you to look at the paper carefully... The paper will change color... It has slowly turned blue... Can you see it?*"

"Yes."

"*It is turning yellow now. Yes, yellow... Can you see?*"

"Yes."

"*It has become red now... Can you see?*"

"Yes."

"*Now the red is going away... It is becoming indistinct... And now you no longer see the color or the paper under it... There is no paper! Can you see the paper?*"

"There's no paper, where's the paper?"

"Yes, the paper has disappeared too… Now your eyelids are getting heavy and they are closing… You are falling into a deeeeep sleep…"

Hypnotizing with a Keyword

If we are going to take the subject under hypnosis multiple times on different days, she could be conditioned with a keyword during her first hypnosis.

"Whenever I say 'Apple' your eyelids will get heavy and you will enter a deep sleep. Now I want you to repeat after me. Whenever I say apple, apple, apple… your eyelids will get heavy and you will enter a deep sleep."

"Whenever you say apple, my eyelids will get heavy and I will enter a deep sleep."

"Whenever I say apple, your eyelids will get heavy and you will enter a deep sleep."

First the hypnotherapist says it, then the subject is asked to repeat, then the hypnotherapist says it one more time.

At the next session, while the subject is sitting in the armchair, she is first asked to take a deep breath and when the therapist says, *"Apple, apple, apple"* he can observe that her eyelids become heavy and that she enters a deep sleep. While the keyword is coded into the subconscious during the session, it is best to code it at the deepest state possible. Because when you repeat the keyword at the next session, you will be receiving the same depth.

After the sessions are completed, the keyword must be removed.

The removal of the keyword will be done under hypnosis, *"From now on, you will not enter a deep sleep whenever I say 'Apple'. The word apple will only remind you of a fruit."*

After the keyword is removed and the subject is taken out of hypnosis, the removal of the suggestion should be double-checked by saying *"Apple, apple, apple."*

Will the subject go into hypnosis if she hears the word apple from someone else other than the hypnotherapist between sessions? No, she will not. It is only connected with your voice tone.

DR. ULUSOY HYPNOSIS INDUCTION TECHNIQUE (Dr. Ulusoy HIT)

It is said that there are as many hypnosis techniques as there are hypnotizers in the World. In my first years, I was using the relatively longer lasting inductions of classical hypnosis such as getting the eyelids heavier and closing them, or collecting the energy of the body starting from the toes to the head and then distributing it to the body as weight.

Later, I developed a technique which is more compatible with the patient, which would not disturb her and would not cause doubt on whether she is in hypnosis or not, and which also eliminates touching. Now I will explain this technique item-by-item.

Dr. Ulusoy Hypnosis Induction Technique

1. Is based on mind – body relaxation,
2. Is focused on auditory – tactile – visual structures,
3. Includes focusing of the eye – breathing – mesmeric hand passing – perception changes, images,
4. Is not disturbing,
5. Contains a pre-evaluation of a couple of minutes, preparation and experience.

Phases of Dr. Ulusoy HIT

A. Auditory

1. She sits toward the edge of the seat with her hands on her knees.
2. She is asked to fix her gaze at the opposite wall, to the intersection of the wall and ceiling.
3. With hand gestures, she is led toward breathing deeply three times and each breath is supported with a positive sentence.
4. At the end of the third breath, she is asked to voluntarily close her eyes.
5. Her eyesight is blocked with the therapist's right hand, creating shadow and a mesmeric pass (Melatonin).
6. She is provided with relaxation suggestions from her head to her neck, to her shoulders, arms, hands, from her neck to her sacrum, to her upper back muscles, her glutes, thighs and legs, and her toes.

7. The suggestion about her body being pulled backwards is given with the magnet-pin example.
8. She is provided with the suggestion, "*When you lean your head and back on the chair, a deep relaxation will reach your body.*"
9. The body will lean on the chair shortly.*

* In case she does not lean back, a voluntary resistance is in question; she is asked to willingly lean her head and back on the chair.

B. Tactile (Perceptual)

1. The suggestion that her left arm has relaxed and become lighter,
2. That her right arm, contrarily, has become heavier like a curbstone or an ingot iron is given.
3. She is asked to provide a yes/no answer to the therapist's question in order to direct him.
4. Do you feel a perceptive difference between your arms? (Y/N)*

* If she doesn't feel any difference in perception, the visual phase should commence.

C. Visual

1. "I want you to imagine a valley between two mountains, in which there are trees, flowers and colorful butterflies. A deep blue stream is flowing splashingly at the bottom of the valley. This is the valley of happiness; you will see, experience, feel and live in this valley of happiness. Now I want you to look around in the valley and tell me about what you see, feel, live and experience."
2. "You have come here to solve an existing problem… Every time you sit in this chair, you will experience a relaxation deeper than the previous one, you will easily receive the suggestions I am giving you, you will smoothly carry out the exercises I will tell you to do, and you will successfully identify yourself with those in the videos that you will watch comfortably, and you will overcome your problem in a short time."

-   If hypnosis is not obtained after the auditory, tactile or visual phases, it means that there is a serious resistance. It could be resulting from excitement, the fear of uncertainty, from the fact that preparations were not sufficient or that the patient has not perceived the preparation, from the fear of losing oneself, or from an obsessive structure -the need to control everything. In such case, a short recess is taken.

- The patient is informed that one or more of these systems will be open in any person, and that she is experiencing this problem because of the anxiety she is having, and because she is not letting herself go. She is told that, in the second exercise, she will directly be receiving suggestions as soon as she sits in the armchair, and she is asked to set her body free as if sitting in a chair at home.
- Some people are unable to imagine things but they can focus their thoughts. Such people are asked to listen to the therapist's words as if listening to a radio theatre.
- An increase in relaxation and suggestibility will be observed in the second session. (Imagination and tactility will open up, or albeit rarely, she will be able to focus her thoughts with her eyes closed.)

She breathes deeply three times and opens her eyes, and she has been evaluated auditorily (+-), tactilely (+-), and visually (+-).

HYPNOSIS DEEPENING TECHNIQUE

Here, I will present you two separate deepening techniques in one single suggestion group. The first one contains energy gathering from the body and distributing it as weight; the second one contains deepening by tiring in dreams during hypnosis and by showing dreams inside dreams. Showing dreams inside dreams provides *dissociation.*

Our subject is in the armchair, preferably in a dark and relatively quiet room at appropriate temperature with an adjustable lighting system directed at the ceiling. These features I have mentioned are not prerequisites. It would be better to have them. It is always important to remember this; if the subject is susceptible, she can easily go into deep hypnosis with a few words, independent of external conditions.

"*Welcome… In this session, I will first take you under hypnosis and then I want to apply additional practices to increase the depth of your hypnosis. As the depth of your hypnosis increases, your conscious enters a separation that we call dissociation. As the result of this dissociation, most of the time, you will* become unaware of what is going on in the outer world. You will only hear my voice and follow it. Depending on the degree of deepening, after I take you out of hypnosis, most probably, you will not remember what we have talked about or what you have experienced during the hypnosis. Your conscious enters these new dissociations -new rooms, so to speak- during hypnosis, and once you come out, the doors of these rooms will have closed. Now, do you allow me to practice this deepening technique on you?"

"Yes."

"Okay, now I am leaning your chair backward. I want you to look at the intersection of the opposite wall and the ceiling. Focus all your attention there. My hand is over your stomach, first you will take a breath and exhale, and my hand will follow your breathing, moving up and down. The rhythm of my hand will be same as your breathing. In the following two breaths, you will follow the up and down movement of my hand with your breathing. You will continue to inhale until my hand reaches the top. You will hold your breath while my hand remains there and you will slowly exhale until my hand reaches all the way down. My hand will wait there for a moment and when I start moving it upwards again, you will start breathing."

"Okay."

(In the meanwhile, I extend my hand toward her abdominal region. I will move it upwards from her stomach and then down again. I will first adjust the height of the movement and its rhythm according to my patient's breathing rhythm. Immediately after that, I will take control of her breathing as her breathing rhythm follows my hand.)

"Take a deep breath. Good, now breathe out... Now take the second breath as you follow my hand... Good. Exhale... Inhale again... Very good. Exhale... As you exhale the third breath, now I want you to close your eyelids with your own wish and will. Yes, very good... From now on, you have shut your eyes with your own wish and will. Your head and neck are gradually loosening and relaxing... Your back and stomach are loosening and relaxing. You are loosening and relaxing from your hips, your thighs, legs and down to your toes... My voice surrounds you all over... There is a great force and energy in our body that moves our organs and muscles. Now I will start from your toes and gather this energy up at your head... This energy is flowing in waves from your toes to your ankles... It is at your ankles now... Can you feel it?"

"Yes."

"Very good. Now I am taking this energy from your ankles to your knees. It *is gaining strength from each point it passes through and it is moving up to your knees. It is at your knees right now... Can you feel it?"*

"Yes."

"Very good. Now I am taking this energy from your knees to your groin. This energy is increasing as it passes through your thighs. It is now at your groin and abdominal region... Can you feel it?"

"Yes."

"This energy has almost caused a whirlpool at your stomach. You start feeling all this energy in your abdominal region that has taken the energy from your lower extremities like a vacuum cleaner... Can you feel it?"

"Yes."

"Good. Now I am taking this energy from your stomach up to your shoulder rotator cuff. The energy coming from your back and chest will join the energy from your stomach and flow toward your rotator cuff. You can also feel the energy flowing from your fingertips to your wrists right now... As it flows from your wrists to your elbows, and from your elbows to your rotator cuff, it joins with all the energy coming from your body... Can you feel it?"

"Yes."

"Now you will feel all the energy of your body at the point on your head where I touch with my thumb... (Press on the top of her head.) *All the energy of your body is flowing toward my thumb... It flows... All the energy of your body is under my control. Your body is weak, tired and exhausted... Now I am going to distribute this energy under my thumb as weights on all over your body. The extremities and body parts that I put weight on will become rock-heavy and you will not be able to move them... First, I am transferring this energy to your eyelids.* (Apply short-term hand passing over the eyelids with your thumb and index finger.) *Your eyelids are as heavy as bullions... Now you can't open them even if you wanted to... You will experience that you can't open them no matter how much you try... Yes, try now... Can you open them?*

(The subject tries to open her eyelids but she cannot.)

"Yes, you see that you cannot open your eyes... Now I will continue to distribute these weights onto your body... I transfer the weight to your neck and shoulders... (Make a hand passing with the palms of both hands over the neck and shoulders from each sides.) *Can you feel this weight on your neck and shoulders?"*

"Yes."

"Very good... Now I am transferring the weight to your arms and hands... (Make a pass starting from the shoulders, over the arms and to the fingertips with both hands.) *Can you feel this weight on your arms and hands?"*

"Yes."

"*Good… Now I am transferring the weight to your back, chest and your abdominal region.* (Make a pass starting from the shoulders to the stomach with both hands. If the therapist is male and the subject is female, this pass is done with the back of the hands, bypassing the chest region.) *Can you feel this weight at your chest and stomach?*"

"Yes."

"*Fine, very good… Now I am transferring this weight to your thighs, legs and down to your toes.* (Again if the therapist is male and the subject is female, do this passing with the back of the hands.) *Now you feel this weight on your legs, right?*"

"Yes."

(If you look carefully, you will see that we took constant feedback while gathering the energy as well as transferring the weight. This feedback helps the subject to be involved and to become deepened with every approval. Step by step, she is experiencing every moment with astonishment.)

"*Youuuuu are sleeeeeping deeeeeply… Youuuuu are sleeeeeping deeeeeply… Youuuuu are sleeeeeping deeeeeply…*"

(Lean toward the subject's right ear and repeat the above sentence three more times. Similarly, lean to her left ear and repeat the sentence three more times. This is the first stage; now we are almost as deep as we wanted to be. Now let's work on increasing the depth some more.)

"*You are in front of an eleven-floor apartment building. On the roof of the building is a person who is about to die. He is fighting for his life. His life depends on you. You have to get him the medicine in your hand as quickly as possible. You will race against time. So, do you want to save him?*"

"Yes."

"*Now start running, run with all your might. You are in the apartment building. The steps are too steep; you started running up. You passed the second floor quickly… You are running to the third floor… You are on the fourth floor… You are getting tired… You are on the fifth floor… You are wearing out… You have arrived at the sixth floor… You feel the tiredness… You have the lofty duty of saving a life… You are at the seventh floor… You are very tired but you go on… You are at the eighth floor… You are exhausted… You are at the ninth floor… Your legs cannot carry you any longer… You are on the tenth floor… You crawl up the remaining stairs… You are on the eleventh floor, on the roof… Right in front of you, you see the dying man. You approach him and give him the medicine in*" *your hand... He drinks and drinks... He is healed and gets on his feet... You feel the joy of having saved a life. But you are really exhausted, aren't you?"*

"Yes."

"You just lie down where you are... Youuuuu are sleeeeeping deeeeeply... Youuuuu are sleeeeeping deeeeeply... Youuuuu are sleeeeeping deeeeeply..."

(We repeat the same suggestion group to both ears, three times each. Let's make it deeper...)

"In this deep sleep, you start dreaming... You are walking in a field with a sweet breeze in springtime... Just ahead, there is a hammock between two trees... With the tiredness of spring, you lie down in the hammock... You go into a deep sleep... Youuuuu are sleeeeeping deeeeeply... Youuuuu are sleeeeeping deeeeeply... Youuuuu are sleeeeeping deeeeeply..."

(We repeat the same suggestion group to both ears, three times each. Let's make it even deeper...)

"In your very deep sleep in the hammock, you have a dream... You are at the seaside in a town by the shore. You lie down on the beach... As you listen to the sounds of waves, you feel the warmth of the Sun... You inhale the smell of iodine from the sea... You are very sleepy... You fall into a deep sleep... Youuuuu are sleeeeeping deeeeeply... Youuuuu are sleeeeeping deeeeeply... Youuuuu are sleeeeeping deeeeeply..."

(We repeat the same suggestion group to both ears, three times each.)

As seen in our deepening pattern, a complete dissociation is provided with,
1. Gathering energy
2. Distributing weights
3. The feeling of helpfulness and tiredness
4. Showing dreams inside dreams (Three dreams)

After this stage, the subject is under deep hypnosis and completely open to suggestion.

SUBCONSCIOUS AND HYPNOSIS

What is The Subconscious anyway?

Every action we initiate with our will (Behaviors, feelings, thoughts) belongs to the conscious. The continuation of the action we have taken voluntarily may again be voluntary, or it could continue under the influence of the subconscious, or it could go on like a blinking lighthouse, between the conscious and the subconscious. We could define the concepts of conscious and subconscious as two rings inside each other... Their boundaries are flexible. This being the case, we perceive it as if we are doing each action at the conscious level. We are mistaken, thinking that there is only one self inside us. Multiple selves, or maybe multiple subconscious elements/shadows guide us. ("There is another I inside me" by Yunus Emre[6], "Ego States" by J. G. Watkins, "Shadows" by Jung.)

The subconscious has the hardware to control emotions, behaviors, thoughts and even the physical body. Where is it located in the brain? We don't know with the information we have as of today... We just say that it is at the right brain and move on.

The Characteristics of the Subconscious that I can Relay According to what I have Read and Observed

1. No time concept
2. No logic
3. No place
4. Contains the principle of equalization
5. Cannot discriminate between dream and reality (Ibn Sina)

Teaching new things to the conscious and to the will is done by observation and training. Teaching things to the subconscious is mostly coincidental. Actually, it would be wrong to say coincidental because the subconscious does not roll the dice, gamble, on the person's mind or body. It has its own principles and conditions of learning. Since we, as humans, don't clearly know its rules, or maybe because we ignore them, the game turns into an absolute gambling...

---

(6)   **TN:** Yunus Emre was a great poet who managed to turn the Anatolian dialect into a language of literature and who succeeded in reciting poetry and chanting hymns in pure Turkish. He has written about issues which looked extremely complex.

The subconscious has two main impulses:
- TO LIVE, provide the continuity of life
- TO REPRODUCE, provide the continuity of the lineage

It eats and drinks, fights, battles for existence in order to live; it is possible to provide more examples... It has strong wishes and desires to reproduce and to continue the lineage... The subconscious is also the intelligent mind.

How does the Subconscious Communicate?

1. Dreams and symbols
2. Freudian slips
3. Gestures and mimics
4. Ideomotor effect
5. Somatization
6. Defense mechanisms such as repression and suppression, introjection, splitting, idealization, devaluation, displacement, steering away, steering to oneself, reflection, identification, projective identification, recreation - formation, denial, isolation, rationalization, dissociation, undoing, intellectualization, concretization, conversion, illusions and dreams, fixation, regression, sublimation... (Defense Mechanisms, Freud)
   Defense mechanisms are structures that protect the ego. They have the purpose of preventing the ego from manifesting itself early -before the true self is formed- and collapsing. All but one –sublimation- appear as pathological but in fact, they are all important to a certain degree.
7. Synchronicity (Jung) and its collective structural connection

How does the Subconscious Learn?

Yes, we may think that it learns by coincidence and that it is like a child who misbehaves all the time. Actually, we are wrong in this idea. Just as *God does not play dice with the universe* (Einstein), the subconscious does not roll dice for the decisions it will take for the mind and body. Therefore, it is more accurate to evaluate the mental and physical illness caused by the subconscious as the process of *faulty learning* (M. Erickson). Okay, but how does the subconscious learn?

In learns through
1. Stories,
2. Anecdotes,

3. Metaphors,
4. Behaviorist traumas,
5. Existentialist wishes and desires.

Its learning is mostly spontaneous.

Information is instilled into the subconscious together with emotions. The individual instillation of the information at the conscious level is called training, education, and emotions don't accompany the information gained in the training at the conscious level.

The fact that stories and metaphors slyly influence the subconscious is due to their indirect approach and effect to the emotional systems.

Since the subconscious does not make reasoning on the decisions it takes and carries out, it cannot think that it could inflict mental or physical harm. For that moment, its decision is correct. For instance, a woman that listens to bad and horrible first night stories cannot be with her husband when she gets married. Her body has spasms, her pupils are dilated, and she pushes her husband away. As the subconscious had not made any reasoning while listening to the negative first night stories, it has done the best thing and locked the system.

Let's see another example; "I have problems to take the penis inside during intercourse, I have contractions. In my dreams, I frequently see myself having normal intercourse with my husband, but suddenly my husband turns me over and forces me for anal sex, and I don't accept it. If he would suggest anal intercourse in real life, I would not accept it. He knows this too," says the woman.

"Dreams are the royal road to the subconscious..." (Freud). Inside the dream, without requiring analysis in the direct sense, the subconscious is presenting the fear regarding the intercourse.

Or a patient, who has taken an appointment for treatment and who is supposed to menstruate one week before the treatment, is late in her menstruation (Even though she is not pregnant) because of the intense fear and emotions she has about the treatment, and she postpones the treatment with the fear of menstruating any time. "My periods always used to be regular, I don't know what happened," she says.

Let's explain what happened; without knowing, she built up her subconscious with her emotion-laden thoughts. And the system delayed her period so that she would stay away from treatment and she would not fear any more. Is the decision taken by the subconscious correct for the moment? Yes. But has it prevented her from being treated? Yes again...

In this case, we need to know how the subconscious system works and how it creates influence, and we need to convey this to our patients. If we could imitate the subconscious' own working principles and interfere with the mind for a short time, we could get one step ahead in healing illnesses.

And the most important advantage of hypnotherapy is that it suspends the conscious and provides easy access to the subconscious.

My medical opinion is that, if we use a method in accordance with the working mechanisms of the subconscious by joining behaviorist treatments with hypnotherapy, we will have taken giant steps toward the healing of mental and physical problems.

THE MIND WORKS WITH MODELLING

Our vaginismus patient's problem was fitting all four models in our quadruple formulation. We began working gradually and with the final session, we arrived at the stage of directing them to intercourse.

During the last session, she said, "Doctor, I had fallen with my bicycle when I was a child and the iron at the middle of the bicycle had struck my genital area, it had hurt a lot. I felt the same pain while doing the exercises you gave me."

Actually, the exercises I had given her were not exercises that could create this pain. But as the mind had been previously coded with a pain attributed to that region, she was perceiving normal exercise touches as that same pain. Although we had worked on her problems in general during hypnotherapy, this link was still in existence.

Our patient was in the session chair and I was standing up, taking notes on the whiteboard. Suddenly I forcefully hit my left hand at the edge of the board in a way that would hurt and also make a sound. Our patient was surprised and she could not understand what was going on. "See," I said, "I felt a severe pain when I hit my hand; it was sharp and agonizing. It still hurts. Then I made a fist with my left hand and I brought my right index finger in and out of the fist. I feel touching and pressure with this action but this is not a real pain like the other one. While doing your exercises, you have the touching feeling as in my second action, but when you had fallen off your bike as a child, you had felt the pain in my first action."

Our patient smiled and said, "You're right."

"The mind works by linking to the past. It thinks and feels as if it would feel the same things, and it creates similar reactions. Let me give you another example. While I was walking past a pastry shop in Nazilli City, I suddenly had a loss of balance and I fell down, hitting my head. When I came around, luckily I was all right. Workups were done at the hospital and no problems were seen. Two weeks passed by, still no problems. While passing by the same pastry shop, I stumbled and almost fell. I took a couple of deep breaths and took shorter steps. I said to myself, "Your mind is playing games with you." I walked by without any problems. If I had panicked at that moment, if I had tried to take precautions with the thought that I would fall again, I would never be able to walk by that pastry shop again. Moreover, my mind would completely take me prisoner in the next stage and I would become unable to even go outside. If we know the working principles of the mind and the subconscious, it becomes easier for us to fight back. Otherwise, we will be in wrong approaches, like Don Quixote attacking windmills."

After that session, our patient went to the hotel with her husband for the experience and they were successful. I asked her after the experience, "Do you still have the same thoughts about the exercises and the experience?"

"No, Doctor," she said, "I understood it very well and I had an easy intercourse."

So, what had I actually achieved with the improvised sudden hitting on the board and the illustration?

This sudden action had created surprise (M. Erickson) and with the surprise, the mental resistances diminished and the mind accepted my illustration. I was able to provide change with improvised manipulation on the patient's mental resistance before taking her under hypnosis.

Many trainees learning hypnotherapy for the first time want to have patterns in their hands. But after learning the rules of the mind and of therapy in the general sense, the rest is your own improvised theatre.

As a psychologist friend of mind once said, "Beyond rules, natural and candid therapy environments can change your patient more easily."

USAGE OF CLINICAL HYPNOSIS IN VAGINISMUS

1. Direct suggestions
2. Indirect suggestions, metaphors, anecdotes
3. Symptom suppression, displacement
4. Autohypnosis
5. Archetypes (Dr. Ulusoy, 2014)
6. Ego Support
7. Imagination
8. Hypnodrama
9. Ideomotor effect and influencing the subconscious
10. Regression
11. Hypnotic relaxation (Whole body relaxation, relaxation with energy gathering – Dr. Ulusoy, 2001)
12. Creating ego state (For today and the future)
13. Utilizing catalepsy
14. Utilizing analgesia and anesthesia
15. Reduction and removal of anxiety
16. Arousal of desire and lust
17. Catharsis and abreaction
18. Muscle stretching and relaxing
19. Simulated muscle stretching and relaxing (Dr. Ulusoy, 2007)
20. Hypothalamus control room technique (Hammond)
21. Seeds planted in thoughts (M. Erickson)
22. The lake archetype
23. Holotropic Breathwork
24. The Hanging Gardens of Babylon (Dr. Ulusoy, 2015)
25. Learning is a process (M. Erickson)
26. The Surprise and Confuse Technique (M. Erickson)
27. The mind learns with modelling (The Honeycomb Model - Dr. Ulusoy, 2006)

Now let's do some suggestion exercises for the above.

1. Direct suggestions

They include directly supporting the ego, creating confidence, convincing her on her capability, and relaxing spasm and supporting patterns.

Example: "*While your mind and body loosen up... You are experiencing this relaxation... You know that everything exists with its contrast... Knowingly or unknowingly, awarely or unawarely, you have inhibited a natural process... You cannot have intercourse... You are afraid, anxious that you will feel pain, you are in panic, worried that it will disrupt, bleed a lot... You think that the vagina is narrow and the penis is too big... You withdraw and have contractions... It is as if you are not yourself at that moment... All the control is out of your hands. You might even think that your willpower has become disabled at that moment...*"

(Up to this point, the body's situation at the moment of intercourse is described to the mind. We are trying to make her subconscious reactions become conscious. We are providing her insight. At the same time, we make the patient realize that we are feeling the same thing as her. First adapt, and then change!)

"*Do you realize that you can see your problem better right now? Yes or no?*

Every person is perfect in essence... As per nature's modus operandi, intercourse and child delivery are normal experiences... You are aware that you cannot remember the normality in your essence because of the wrong information you have learned in life... (Faulty learnings, M. Erickson)

From now on, you know that every area in your body is relaxing... If you want, let's tighten your extremities one by one... First your left hand; let it tighten up and become stiff... Can you feel the stiffness at your left hand? Yes or no?

Now let your right hand tighten up and become stiff... Can you feel the stiffness at your right hand? Yes or no?

Now let your left foot tighten up and become stiff... Can you feel the stiffness at your left foot? Yes or no?

Now let your right foot tighten up and become stiff... Can you feel the stiffness at your right foot? Yes or no?

You have experienced the tightening and stiffening of your extremities one by one... You are aware that you have control over all your muscle groups. When you lie in bed to have intercourse, you will easily be able to move your legs down, up, right and left... You will let your partner approach, place the penis at the vagina entrance... While adapting to its kind but firm structure and to its specific heat with relaxation, your breathing will be comfortable and rhythmical... You will reach the awareness that you are not feeling pain, that you feel touching and pressure, and that the possible pain at the hymen is easily tolerable..."

2. Indirect suggestions, metaphors, anecdotes

"Look, if I place a wooden plank on the floor and ask you to walk on it, you could easily with your eyes open or closed. If I put that plank between the roofs of two five-floor buildings, you could not dare to walk on the same plank you just walked on. Pain is a relative concept. After coming home and changing after a busy schedule during the day, you must have had times when you had seen a bruised spot on your body, one that you don't remember hitting anywhere and one that you wonder how it hadn't made you feel any pain... So from now on, you will not feel pain or ache during the intercourse..."

"With our hands and fingers, we can do detailed and fine work. We can write, use a keyboard, or knit. There are different muscle groups on our fingers and these muscle groups work in coordination with each other to help us do the finely detailed works. The same muscle groups also exist at your back, your hips, your vagina and your legs. So from now on, your back muscles, hip muscles, vagina muscles and your leg muscles will start working in coordination and concordance with each other..."

3. & 4. Symptom displacement and Autohypnosis

These are mostly used instrumentally in further stages. If the contractions have been reduced but are still ongoing in a way that prevents intercourse despite the given suggestions, the contractions at the legs could be transferred to a more convenient place, to the arm or fist, for example.

"From now on, I want you to think about and feel the final moment of the experience. I want you to feel the same tension in your legs as you had felt it at that moment... Yes, can you feel this tension and strain? Yes or no?

Now I will transfer this tension and strain to your left hand... First, I want you to make a fist with your left thumb left inside... Good, just like that... Now as your legs gradually relax, the contraction moves to your left fist.... I can see the tension in your fist... You can feel it... At the time of intercourse, I will make a fist with my left thumb inside... I will say the number 747 three times in a row, 747, 747, 747... As my left hand makes a fist with a strong contraction, my back muscles, hip muscles, vagina muscles and my leg muscles will loosen up even further... Now I want you to repeat after me... I will say the number 747 three times in a row, 747, 747, 747... As my left hand makes a fist with a strong contraction, my back muscles, hip muscles, vagina muscles and my leg muscles will loosen up even further... Okay, very good... Now we repeat one more time... I will repeat the number 4 three times in a row, 747, 747, 747... As my left hand makes a fist with a strong contraction, my back muscles, hip muscles, vagina muscles and my leg muscles will loosen up even further..."

With this technique, the existing contraction is transferred to the left fist. Sometimes the contraction is so strong that it could reach the left arm or even the shoulder. After the penis experience is realized, symptom displacement is not really necessary for other experiences.

This is also an autohypnosis technique in a way. Symptom Displacement and Autohypnosis have been used together.

5. Archetypes (Dr. Ulusoy, 2014)

Going to the Source – The River Motif: "*You are in front or a river. But the river is flowing slowly and weakly... You decide to go to the water's source. While you walk toward the spring, you see the debris and rocks in front of the water. You have reached the spring... What is that? The spring is very weak and gauntly. You have all the tools and equipment you need. Now you are widening the spring. The water is flowing affluently now. Good... But you don't settle with this. You open up a new spring with the tools you have. The waters from both springs have joined and the water flow has become immense. It is overflowing to the riverbed... Now you follow the water. The water passes over all the obstacles and debris in its way, it is sweeping them along... You have reached the point, the delta where the river meets the sea. In happiness and joy, you are experiencing the uniting of the river and the sea...*"

It is a suggestion that uses subconscious resources and that contains the joining of the river and the sea at the delta (Vagina) without focusing on the problem, via an archetype.

The Hero's Journey: "*You have bothers about your problem which you haven't been able to solve... You have moved away from people in order to see your problems, fight with them and to find solutions... You are in front of a cave... It is pitch-dark inside... You are holding a torch and a sharp sword... You enter the cave... When you go down one level, oh God, what is that? There is a seven-headed dragon... You are anxious at first but then you decide to fight it... As you swing your sword masterfully, each of the dragon's heads fall down with each blow... 1...2...3...4...5...6...7... Yes... The dragon is neutralized now.... You pass it by and go down six more levels under the earth... There is a chest in the room you have arrived at... You slowly open the lid of the chest... You find a letter written personally for you and specific to your problem... You take it out of the chest and read in the light of the torch... When your reading is finished, I want you to inform me by lifting your left index finger... Okay, now you declared* that your reading is over... The information you have received there belongs only to you and to your problem... With this information, you climb up the levels... You have arrived at the cave entrance... Now you can return home with this new information and experience..."

This is again a suggestion that is not focused on the problem and that is designed for her to create her own solution.

6. Ego Support

"You are a self-confident individual with her feet firmly on the ground... You were not aware of your power until now... You saw yourself as weak, helpless and pitiful in your intercourse trials... But you have done great things ever since you were born... You were a tiny baby... You were crawling... Then you wanted to stand up, to be liberated... You fell in your first try... Because your ankles were not developed enough and they could not carry you. When your ankles developed, you fell once more before even taking a few steps. Your knee joints had not develop enough... When your knee joints developed, you increased your number of steps but you fell once again... Because your hip joint had not developed... But today, you can easily walk and run... You learned how to walk, despite all obstacles, and you did not refrain from trying to walk, from being liberated... Walking requires learning. So, from now on, you can learn how to have intercourse with the awareness of the strong ego inside yourself..."

This is a suggestion technique that supports the ego and that can also be used to remind learning.

7. Imagination & Simulation

"Imagination exists in humans. Not only can this imagination heal illnesses, it can also create illnesses out of nothing." (Ibn Sina)

The mind cannot differentiate between reality and imagination. Both reality and imagination stimulate the same neurons at the same part of the brain. From this mutual point, the imaginations under hypnosis are very valuable. In a sense, imaginations can be used as simulations.

"You are with your husband in a convenient moment... You and your husband desire each other very much... You closely feel your husband's warmth, his skin and his breath... While planting small kisses on each other, your lust and desire grow... You feel your skin, your body loosens up and you get wet... You are focused only on the moment you are living in... You don't think of the past or the future... For you, there is only the NOW... While living this moment, you leave yourself into the pleasure... As you take off your clothes one by one, you have left yourself completely to the moment and to the flow... Like a paper boat sailing with the water current... You experience your husband's penis touch the outside of your genitalia and you get wetter... You slowly place your husband's penis between your vaginal lips and you experience its warmth... You trust your husband and believe him... Without even knowing it, you feel your husband slipping his penis from your vaginal lips to the vagina, giving you a sweet warmth and fullness... As you embrace your husband, you experience him going in and out... While you feel the kind but firm touch, the pressure and the warmth, you also feel the pleasure more intensely... When your husband ejaculates, you also experience pleasure in all your body with small trembles..."

8. Hypnodrama

"We imagine a theatre stage. All the seats in front of the stage are empty... You sit at the seat that has the best view of the stage... The curtain is pulled open in both directions... The light illuminates the left side of the stage. What is that? Your look-alike appears at the left side of the stage. It is your ego that is weak, helpless, unable to have intercourse, withdrawing, scared and contracting... Now the light moves to the right side of the stage... Here is another look-alike but she is coming with firm steps in self-confidence. It is your ego that can do the exercises (This is a suggestion recommended for use after finger exercises) easily, and that will have a smooth intercourse with pleasure... While both of your egos look at you from the middle of the stage, your ego from the left side starts to speak, 'I have protected and looked after you until now. I can also protect you from now on.'

Then the strong ego takes the floor, 'Yes, knowingly or not, you have created her but I am also inside you. I am your strong ego that will have a smooth intercourse and take pleasure in doing so. You met me just today..."

The helpless ego steps back in, 'Why would you believe her? If you were a strong ego as you claim to be, wouldn't you have had this intercourse earlier?'

The strong ego replies, 'If you can't see the Sun on a cloudy day, if you can't see the stars when you look up to the sky in the morning, you still can't deny that they are there. Just as you can't deny them, you can't deny me either. I was always inside of you... You just noticed me today...'

As both egos continue to look at you, you walk up to the stage... You take your helpless and weak ego down from the stage... Not only do you take her down but you also escort her to the door of the hall... Not only do you escort her to the door of the hall, you also walk next to her up to the main gate of the theatre building... You look at her one last time, and see her off with the awareness of *knowing that you don't need her anymore... When she completely moves away, when she disappears in the horizon and when you are no longer able to see her, you go back in from the gate and lock it tightly from the inside... Even if she did come back accidentally, she cannot come in from the gate. Now you walk to the hall and you also lock the door of the hall tightly from the inside... Now that stage and that strong ego on it belong to you... You run toward your strong ego, embrace her and become one..."*

9. Ideomotor effect and influencing the subconscious

"I want you to raise both hands as if you are praying... Elbows up, arms close to each other... Now I want you to think about your problem...the moments when you feel scared, unable to have intercourse... While you think about these, I am looking for a symbol to describe this problem... Yes, I want you to think of a rectangle... I am placing this rectangle onto your left palm as a symbol of the problem... The symbol of the problem is in your left palm... Now I am looking for an internal source for this problem...an internal source that solely belongs to this problem and that can solve this problem... Yes, I want you to think of a prism... I am placing this prism onto your right palm as the symbol of internal source... The problem symbol is in your left palm, and the internal source is in your right palm... Now, with your will and under my observation, if the subconscious is able to solve the existing problem with its own internal source, your hands will come together and touch each other like the opposite poles of the magnet attracting one another..."

The hands will gradually come closer and touch each other with the *saw tooth* movement, which is an action of the subconscious. It could be completed in two or three minutes, but there have been cases that reach up to twenty minutes. The therapist needs to wait patiently. If necessary, *directed imagination* could be done with suggestions. In such direction-giving, the energies on both sides of the body may be gathered and transferred to the hands. Or external energy transfer could also be done. In rare cases, it is seen that the hands do not meet, or that they move even further apart. In this case, the therapist should consider an unresolved situation about the problem in the subconscious, or a situation that has not been revealed to the physician by the patient, such as molestation or rape.

Providing subconscious interaction of the problem with the internal sources with the ideomotor effect via the hands is an application of Dr. Albert Schmierer. The ideomotor definition belongs to M. Erickson.

10. Regression

Regression means taking back to an earlier age. The patient is taken from her actual age gradually to her moment of birth, and investigation is done on whether there is a cause for the problem. There may be multiple causes that are spread over time. As in the Coex Systems of S. Grof, structures that contain similar emotions experienced in the past may trigger the illness.

The Coex Systems are interesting in the way that they harbor similar emotions inside themselves. Such that; in most of vaginismus patients, there are commonly seen reactions, feelings of pain and fear that are against blood, needles, insects, swimming, driving, etc. The interesting part is that, although we do not work on such fears during vaginismus treatment, I receive feedback from most patients after treatment, informing me that other fears have also been eliminated. And this supports S. Grof's Coex Systems.

In regression, the ego has to be supported with suggestions while each event related to the problem is being relived. Actually, the therapist does not have much influence in this process. Since the event experienced in the past could not be solved with the consciousness state at the time, it has been pushed into the subconscious, and the subconscious creates the defensive reaction of today. During regression, the patient re-encounters the material pushed into the subconscious. While the event is being experienced once more with the current state of consciousness, the conscious and the subconscious gain insight. The event that has been experienced with the current state of consciousness becomes freed of the burden of emotion; it has become a memory that is plain and available for erasure. This situation is also the process that Freud calls "Abreaction and catharsis – Chimney cleaning."

The event is evaluated with the current level of consciousness, and it is also cleansed of the emotional burdens because it has been relived with all the related emotions.

I would like to provide a couple of examples for this.

Example 1: While our patient is sitting at the dinner table in her high school years, her father dashes in and slaps his daughter fiercely for no reason and says, "So you're going to be a whore like your cousin, is that right?" The girl has not understood anything; involuntarily the slap has coded pain, prostitution and intercourse into the subconscious. Before coming home, the father had found out about her cousin's forbidden relationship with a man, and he had reacted fiercely at his daughter. Unfortunately, that girl, who was not aware of anything, appeared before us as a vaginismus patient. *The shock and the following sentence* had made a strong suggestive effect.

Example 2: Her grandmother had taken off the underpants of the girl, who had been late to complete her toilet training, and lit a match to threaten the girl, saying, "Will you ever wet yourself again?"

Regression and the moment of birth

When we further continue regression, we reach the mother's womb. We can make the patient feel and relive the situation of the baby in her mother's womb. As the patient experiences the feeling that her needs are being met and the feeling of a peaceful environment, it could be useful to use suggestions to transfer this peace and comfort to the moment of intercourse after the regression.

At the same time, the patient, who experiences the moment of birth (Normal delivery), re-experiences the fact that her own head can pass through the vagina channel. This way, she relives the feeling that the vagina is elastic and gains insight on the fact that the penis could fit in there.

Previous lives in regression

Is there such a thing as previous life, or not? Do we come to Earth just once? Or is the karma mechanism in effect? Or are previous lives just fantasies of the subconscious? Or do they originate from Jung's collective subconscious?

While dropping anchor in your mind with these questions, I would like to talk about a vaginismus case related to a scenario of a previous life.

Example: She experienced living in the Medieval Age, in a rattrap by the stream. She was not doing well financially. She was overweight and dirty. There were about ten kids around her and they were all hers. She was not able to look after herself or her children. The fathers of the children were unknown; there was no father in the picture. She was having affairs with multiple men.

I asked her if this situation was bothering her. She said that it did. I took her further back in her life and made her experience being born in a nice house and a rich family. As I continued to make her experience her marriage to a rich and handsome man when she came to the age of marriage, I also made her experience having two children that they could easily look after.

Afterwards, I continued the age regression and took her to her mother's womb first, and then to her current age before ending the session.

The data on the previous life had caused her trilogy of *marriage = ugliness + poverty + too many children to take care of.* And this was the underlying reason of her vaginismus. After this exercise, the patient's contractions disappeared and she had the intercourse experience.

11. Hypnotic relaxation

As in many mental diseases, the main factors in sexual problems are stress, anxiety, fear, panic and contractions. Hypnotic relaxation is more effective that standard relaxation. In standard relaxation, each muscle group -from the head to the toes- is first stretched and strained, and then relaxed. Whereas in clinical hypnosis, even taking your patient in and out of induction is perceived as relaxation.

12. Creating ego state

Ego states are actually Dr. Watkins' theory in hypnotherapy. While using this in clinical hypnosis, we make the patient imagine the problematic ego of today and the ego of the future that has overcome the problem. While the characteristics of today's problematic ego are made indistinct, the future-expected ego with positive features is made more active. The distancing of the helpless ego and the creation of the strong ego in hypnodrama is another example of creating ego state.

13. Utilizing catalepsy

Arm catalepsy is created in patients with erectile dysfunction or premature ejaculation problems. Afterwards, this catalepsy is supported with a keyword and with the imagination technique for transferring it to the erection state. With the given keyword, the person can control his erection or premature ejaculation during intercourse.

14. Utilizing analgesia and anesthesia

It can especially be used against vaginal sensitivity in vaginismus treatment. It would also be appropriate to use it in premature ejaculation to create a temporary numbness at the tip of the penis. Firstly a pain-free region at the back of the hand is created with suggestion. A needle is stuck to the back of the hand both during hypnosis and also after the patient gets out of hypnosis, while the pain-free region is still in effect. The patient experiences that the needle is being stuck in her hand without any feeling of pain, both in and out of hypnosis. Afterwards, this pain-free region is carried to our desired area with suggestions, and its usage is conditioned with a keyword. A model has been created at the back of the hand and then the created model has been carried elsewhere. The mind learns with models.

15. Reduction and removal of anxiety

Anxiety is the feeling of worry, fear and distress by thinking that something bad will happen to us, even when there is no possibility of such event. Control of the anxiety may be provided by applying hypnotic systemic desensitization, hypnotic relaxation, or breathing control exercises.

16. Arousal of desire and lust

In sexual problems, desire and lust may be missing from the start, or desire and lust may be reduced due to sexual problems encountered. In both processes, clinical hypnosis is effective in the arousal of desire and lust. This is provided with imagination and simulation. You may read suggestion patterns on this in further pages.

17. Catharsis and abreaction

Actually, Freud had noticed two very important things during the years he used hypnosis in therapy: Catharsis and abreaction. While these two structures were creating discharge via emotions, they were also providing therapeutic healing in the patient. But he was worried about the transfer so he developed free verbal association. His aim in free verbal association was to render the subconscious conscious. This step that he took caused the abandonment of catharsis and abreaction which were the healing tools for man's intelligent mind. In fact, these were some lost years for psychotherapists. Today, psychiatry evaluates catharsis and abreaction as healers in post-traumatic stress syndrome, and it is curious why it has slandered this approach in other problems...

Other than psychosomatic diseases, you are also familiar with psychoneuroimmunology. The underlying factor in psychosomatic diseases is the negative effect of suppressed emotions on the body. Such emotions, which have been suppressed for being deemed dangerous at the time, cannot be sorted out by the conscious, and during the period in which they are not sorted out, they are not allowed to go up to the conscious level because they are deemed dangerous by the subconscious. The subconscious uses intensive energy to maintain its suppressive defense. It sucks the energy out of the body like a vacuum. Therefore, local and/or general weakening and blockages are formed in the body's energy system. These emotions that are suppressed with decreasing energy and blockages also effect the immune system. While being in constant contact with microorganisms everywhere, infections develop only in case the defense mechanism of the immune system is weakened due to malnutrition and/or emotional suppressions.

Consequently, utilizing intelligent mind in therapy, rather that verbal therapy, will provide the removal of these blockages and the holistic health of the mind-body. At the same time, as I have mentioned under the regression topic, it will be helpful in being freed from the emotional burden of the event if the patient in vaginismus treatment can relive the event in her current consciousness level and gain insight.

18. Muscle stretching and relaxing

Another way to remove the contractions experienced during intercourse is the muscle stretching and relaxing exercises. In practice, this situation is done, also without hypnosis, by the patient lying on her back and stretching and releasing her muscle groups one by one, starting from her neck to her toes. The aim is to experience contractions consciously and then to learn relaxation.

It provides positive and much better results to apply the same process to each separate muscle group with suggestions under hypnosis.

19. Simulated muscle stretching and relaxing (Dr. Ulusoy, 2007)

Under hypnosis, the patient thinks about the moment of intercourse and she is asked to feel the same contraction in her legs as it happens at that moment. Tension starts at the patient's legs. First, the tension and contraction are moved to the right leg and the left leg is loosened up with suggestion. Then, the tension and contraction is moved to the left leg, and both legs are loosened up with suggestion. After that, the tension and contraction are moved to the right arm, and both legs and the left arm are loosened up with suggestion. The tension and contraction are translocated... They disappeared while relocating... *"A tension and contraction that is able to relocate does not belong to that region of yours, but they belong to your mind... So, you could experience a comfortably intercourse without tension or contraction..."* Here, a strong suggestion is given via the body to the subconscious insinuating, "See, it is not physical; you can let it go if it belongs to you..."

20. Hypothalamus control room technique (Hammond)

This technique is practiced by making the patient imagine that there is a control room in the brain. We can use this technique for the following.
i.   Removing vaginal pain

ii.   Providing ability to touch the vagina and reducing the feeling of pressure

iii. Premature ejaculation

iv.   Erectile dysfunction

In this technique, under hypnosis, the person enters the control room in the brain. She sits at the chair in front of the instrument panel inside the control room. On the panel, there is a key system that is numbered from one to ten. The patient is asked to say at which level -from one to ten- her existing problem stands. According to the received answer, this level is decreased or increased gradually in separate sessions.

During the exercises in vaginismus, the level at the panel is decreased from ten to one to reduce vaginal pain, vagina touching problem and the feeling of pressure. The level at the panel is increased from one to ten to prolong the duration in premature ejaculation, or to provide erection in erectile dysfunction.

The entrance to the control room is done through an encoded door. The patient is given suggestions that no one else but she can enter. She enters with the code and comes out with the code.

21. Seeds planted in thoughts (M. Erickson)

During the years when I had not yet reduced the treatment period to one and a half days, we had worked primarily on hypnotherapy with my patient that had come from abroad. But as our time was limited, they were not able to experience the intercourse fully. Her contractions were ongoing.

During hypnosis, I asked my patient to imagine two hills. The first hill was a rocky and barren place, while the other hill was filled with green fields and butterflies. I told her that she was currently on the arid, barren and rocky hill, and that she somehow had to pass to the green hill where she wanted, desired to be, to live on.

I told her she had three ways.

i.   You can hang a wire between the hills and you can slide on this wire to pass across.

ii.   You can come down the hill and climb the other one.

iii. You can call a helicopter and go across in the helicopter.

"What would you like to do?" I asked.

After giving it some thought, the patient said, "I'm calling a helicopter." She got on the helicopter and landed on the other hill. She was very happy.

I ended the session. I asked her to try intercourse when they went home and to inform me via e-mail. They did not get back to me during the following week. On Sunday evening, she wrote, "Thank you, we experienced the intercourse, we made it."

Behind the success was an interesting synchronicity (i.e. Jung – The story of the scarab).

She had refrained from trying intercourse during the week because she was nervous. On Sunday morning, she got out to the garden, arranging her flowers. She saw the helicopter bug flying among her flowers. She suddenly remembered the suggestion about the helicopter during hypnosis. And she ran home, woke up her husband and told him that she wanted to have sex, and then she had a comfortable intercourse while she and her husband looked at each other in bafflement.

What kind of a mechanism was in place here? The indirect suggestion, which was left inside a closed box in the mind as a metaphor, was opened later after being triggered by an external stimulus and it eliminated the problem.

22. The lake archetype

Catathymia: Also called *Spiritual Image Experience*, it is a therapy that is applied to a relaxed body with closed eyes. We could also call it the imagination stage of hypnosis. It was founded and applied by the German Psychiatrist Leuner. In fact, the themes in catathymia belong to Jung's psychology.

If the patient has worries, fears, repulsions regarding sexuality, or if she has experienced incest, molestation, rape in the past, she may say that the lake is dirty, unclear or slimy when she is asked to imagine a lake under hypnosis.

If you pay attention, the subconscious is as tight-lipped as it is in dreams. It conveys the existing problem via symbols.

If we follow my own therapy theory, we need to make arrangements and changes in the lake archetype via symbolization and by using the symbol given by the subconscious to reverse engineer the working mechanism of the subconscious.

Firstly, if there are channels that pollute the dirty and slimy lake, we either block them or change their course, and then we provide clean water sources to flow into the lake. Then we use special equipment to remove the dirty and slimy water out of the lake, making the patient visualize the lake getting cleaner and clearer. The lake becomes so clean that our patient can see the fish swimming in it even by looking from the outside. Even the ducks swimming on the water...

We have used this technique on one of our vaginismus patients, and after the therapy, she had expressed her feelings of great inner peace and relaxation. Her problem was solved in the following sessions.

23. Holotropic Breathwork

It may be used on patients whose resistant contractions continue despite therapy.

Holotropic Breathwork was founded by Psychiatrist S. Grof. After his altered conscious state studies that he carried out with LSD (A strong synthetic narcotic drug), he realized that breathing could also alter consciousness, same as LSD.

The patient lying on her back is asked to close her eyes. She is supported to breathe deeply but more rapidly. Even if one may think that breathing rapidly and deeply supplies more oxygen for the brain, in fact, this is a paradox. Actually, there is no increased oxygen but the carbon dioxide starts to increase in the brain. And the increase in carbon dioxide causes metabolic alkalosis. This type of breathing causes the cortex (The top shell of the brain), i.e. the conscious, to be suppressed.

After a certain time, images from the subcortical archaic structures start to appear in replacement for the suppressed subconscious. Actually, this is a form of trance. At the same time, numbness starts at the extremities and spreads to various parts of the body. According to Grof, in a sense, the individual in this state is having a spiritual crisis and this crisis is supported by the therapist next to him. The therapist is an observer in this situation. As the situation suppressed in the subconscious surfaces, the patient reevaluates the event with her current consciousness level and she is freed of the burden of the suppressed emotion. The experienced situation could be the surfacing of a real event that had been pushed into the subconscious in the past, or it could be a scenario created by the subconscious. After this therapy that goes on with archaic images and reactions via the body, a general relaxation and loosening is observed at the patient.

It could be used as a supplementary technique for the contractions of a resistant vaginismus patient.

24. The Hanging Gardens of Babylon (Dr. Ulusoy, 2015)

It is a sample of a mythological, modified, metaphorical story that is given to the vaginismus patient during the first session according to the 5-BK Model. It will also be used to enrich the description of the stages during the following sessions.

"The Hanging Gardens of Babylon are one of the World's Seven Wonders...

Now together with you, we want to create the World's eighth wonder that belongs to you. Imagine a five-floor historical structure like a pyramid with a wide base that narrows as it goes upwards, and which has garden terraces at each floor. At the fifth floor, there is a pink-painted house that portrays happiness with its white louvers and smoking chimney, and with the joyous sounds of children inside the house.

Now you are in front of this five-floor structure, at the ground level. And you want to reach the top where there is the house that you desire, that you want to live in, with its pink-paint, white louvres, smoking chimney and happy children's sounds, and whose door is opened fully for you.

There are five doors that lead to each floor. You open the door in front of you. You close the first door from the inside and lock it, never to return there again. You throw the key out over the wall. The garden on this floor is full of wild flowers. Daisies and tulips spring out from among the green grass... You can feel the smell of the daisies and the grass as you walk in the garden... This place gets you into a sweet excitement and motivation... If it is so beautiful here, who knows how beautiful the next floor is, and how much more it will motivate you.

You reach the stairs that lead to the second floor and you open the door in front of you to enter the second garden... You close and lock the door, never to return. You throw the key out over the wall. There are hyacinths and daffodils in this garden... As you walk among them happily and peacefully, you feel the wonderful scent of the hyacinths and daffodils reaching the depths of your body... If it is so beautiful here, who knows how beautiful the next floor is, and how much more it will motivate you.

You walk up the stairs to the third floor and you open the third door to enter the third garden. You close and lock the door, never to return. You throw the key out over the wall. There are lavenders and jasmines all around... The beautiful flower scents come to you in the form of peacefulness... If it is so beautiful here, who knows how beautiful the next floor is, and how much more it will motivate you.

You walk up the stairs to the fourth floor and open the fourth door to enter the fourth garden... You close and lock the door, never to return. You throw the key out over the wall. In this garden, there are lilacs and magnolias. Inside, you feel the color harmony of the lilacs and magnolias and their magnificent smells... If it is so beautiful here, who knows how beautiful the next floor is, and how much more it will motivate you.

You are about to reach the top floor... You have a sweet tranquility and excitement inside. You go up the stairs that lead to the fifth floor and you open the fifth door in front of you and walk into the garden... You close and lock the door, never to return. You throw the key out over the wall. There are roses in various colors in this garden... White, yellow, red, light pink...so many colors... They smell wonderful... Nightingales are singing among the roses... You can hear them... A bit further you enter the house with pink-paint, white louvres, a smoking chimney and in which you hear the sounds of the happy laughters and happiness of parents and children...

Now this house belongs to you and your husband... You will now live here with joy, health, peace, sexual happiness and pleasure for as long as you want..."

25. Learning is a process (M. Erickson)

In the 5-BK Model, if the patient could not open one of the doors, or if she has opened it halfway, the following learning story should be presented under hypnosis.

"Do you remember your infanthood? If any of your relatives has a baby or if you have a younger sibling, have you watched them go through their crawling and walking stages? Babies are curiously inclined to learning. First, they want to crawl out of their environment to better see what is going on around them... After crawling, they want to rise on their feet but they fall because their ankles are not developed enough... When their ankles are developed, they try to stand up but they fall again because their knee joints are not fully developed... After their knee joints are developed, they are able to take a few steps but they fall again because their hip joints are not developed enough... Despite all these failures and all the pain they suffer with each fall, they don't lose any motivation and finally they learn how to walk...

Don't forget that you were also a baby once... Now you don't even think about how you are able to walk...

So, you can use your inner resource of success that exists in your subconscious to open the door that you could not open/ or half-open, and to pass to the next step...

26. The Surprise and Confuse Technique (M. Erickson)

This technique has been inspired by the story of Erickson helping J. Zieg to give up smoking. It could be given as suggestions under hypnosis. The construction belongs to me. It helps the mind to be confused with different schemes against the fear and contractions schemes of the intercourse that the mind is expecting. And this provides the intercourse to be experienced more easily, without even knowing it. Below is an example from one of my hypnosis sessions.

"I had a patient... She was wondering if she could have intercourse with her

husband or not... Was she going to have sex at home or in a hotel? Was she going to be comfortable during sex or nervous? Was she going to prefer a position that she was on top or at the bottom? Was she going to look at her husband's penis or was she going to close her eyes? Was she going to wrap her legs around her husband or was she going to lie flat? Was she going to pull her legs to her stomach or was she going to lean them on her husband's shoulders? Was she going to feel her husband's penis touching the entrance of her vagina or feel one-thirds of it inside? Was she going to feel one-thirds of it inside or half? Was she going to feel half of it enter or all of it? Was she going to feel all of it entering or going out? Was she going to feel it go out or the pumping motion inside? Was she going to feel the warmth of her husband's penis or the warmth when her husband ejaculates? Was she going to feel pleasure before her husband or was her husband going to feel the pleasure first?"

27. The mind learns with modelling
(The Honeycomb Model - Dr. Ulusoy, 2006)

The mind learns with modelling. Therefore, you need to make a point of creating models while forming your suggestion patterns... Knowledge on its own does not provide learning. The mind founds the information on the patterns that it has from the past, or on the new patterns that you present. This is just like providing bees with a comb for them to make honey.

Let's read the example together.

"With our hands and fingers, we can do detailed fine work. We can write, use a keyboard. There are different muscle groups on our fingers and these muscle groups work in coordination with each other to help us do the finely detailed works. The same muscle groups also exist at your back, your hips, your vagina and your legs. So from now on, your back muscles, hip muscles, vagina muscles and your leg muscles will start working in coordination and concordance with each other...

If I place a wooden plank on the floor and ask you to walk on it, you could easily with your eyes open or closed. If I put that plank between the roofs of two five-floor buildings, you would be nervous and you would refrain from walking on the same plank you just walked on. What have changed are the mental sets and obstacles. So from now on, all your mental sets and obstacles preventing you from having intercourse are being removed one by one...

Pain is a relative concept. After coming home and changing after a busy schedule during the day, you must have had times when you had seen a bruised spot on your body... And you immediately wonder where you hit it and why you didn't feel any pain... Pain is a relative concept... So from now on, you will not feel pain or ache during your dildo exercises or during the penis stage ...

You were raised with negative stories in the past, experienced sexual traumas, and at the same time, you -or your parents- developed a protective instinct. Now the emotions of all this are turning into an indistinct, pale picture for you. As the picture turns pale and indistinct, even if you remember the events, they will not bother you as they did before... As a small child, perhaps you needed a protective instinct but with your current age and mental level, you are able to prevent any external abuse...

And you will have this relationship, not to make your husband happy or to satisfy your longing for motherhood, but for your own physical happiness and pleasure. Afterwards, your husband's happiness will come, and at a later time of your choosing, your longing for motherhood will come to an end. So, from today on, you will have comfortable intercourse, knowing that you are on legal grounds with your husband...

If we were to liken the outer and inner vaginal lips to an animal, perhaps we could liken them to a cute rabbit with long ears... Imagine that you move toward the rabbit, that you touch it, that it leans on your chest and shoulder, and that you feel its warmth and softness...

While you live in an arid, barren and rocky place, your journey to the place that you wish, you desire and that you want to live in continues. Even if you face small problems during this journey, you feel the strength and courage inside you to overcome all of them... You are seeing and experiencing the fact that we have cut your mountain-like problem into small pieces, and as we approach each piece you see that it is nothing more than an anthill...

And a vagina has a structure that is capable of taking in any length or diameter of a dildo or penis whether it is long or short, large or small. And you reach the awareness that you, as a woman, have such a vagina... Your right hip and left leg loosen up... Your left hip and right leg loosen up... When you want to have sex with your husband, you will be able to move your legs up and down, right and left easily. You will feel your husband placing his penis at the vagina entrance, and its sweet but firm stiffness, and its specific warmth...

In order to take your husband's penis in, like a seagull diving into water, standing on the water and then flapping its wings to glide to the sky, you respond to his leaning motion with your mental and physical relaxation. You will easily let your husband come in, to go out and to move inside you... You will have the best sex with your husband for the rest of your life, whenever you want, wherever you want and in whichever position you want."

HYPNOSIS AND PAIN CONTROL

Perhaps the most impressive part of hypnosis is the removal of pain. It includes visible, almost palpable and astonishing visuality and experience. It has a wide range, from sticking a needle at the back of the hand to major surgeries, and it can be experienced either under hypnosis or with posthypnotic suggestions when awake.

Pain control is an almost magical application that helps individuals under hypnosis to understand that they are in hypnosis and that they are receiving suggestions. It is surprising, spectacular and magical.

Within medicine and psychology sciences, mechanisms that are still not exactly defined play a part in pain control. And it is still surprising, spectacular and magical for therapists, too.

This situation is more than blocking the nerve impact areas (Dermatomes) with anesthetic substances; it is an anesthesia that includes the areas that you have drawn from the outside. The pain signal that reaches the cortex is perceived by the cortex as painlessness. Our brain is constructed on models, exemplifications and experiences. Since the brain cannot differentiate reality and imagination -because it responds to both as real- cognitive distortions, negative emotional ascribing and stories can also lower or heighten pain threshold.

The best example for this situation is the cognitive distortions we see in vaginismus patients. It will hurt a lot, bleed a lot, my eyes will be locked on the ceiling when the penis enters, something like an iron chair leg or a broomstick is going to enter, etc. etc. These emotion-laden sentences create new models in the brain that lower the pain threshold. This situation prevents intercourse and it also causes patients to have a higher sensation of the pain that is felt during the penetration of something (Dilator during pre-exercises or penis in the next stages).

As seen, the mechanism works both ways. The felt pain can be reduced or eliminated with hypnotic suggestions, and it can be increased unknowingly with emotions or stories.

What a nice system we have been given at birth; it is possible for us to go into the control room and play with the adjustments, to create changes in favor of our health.

There were a few paragraphs in the new book *The Book of Pain* released by Hayy Publishing and written by Dr. Serdar Erdine, who has had serious non-hypnotic studies on pain.

"Ibn Sina has defined pain in fifteen types; scratching, stiffness feeling, constricting, puckering, breaking, soft, piercing, stinging, numbing, pulsating, heavy feeling, tiring and burning pain."

I think these descriptions are important because they allow us to describe the pain that we want to remove under hypnosis and also to increase the effectiveness of the suggestion. What kind of pain is our patient feeling? It will make things easier if we define the pain she feels and provide her with suitable suggestions. (Dr. Ulusoy)

Again, Melzack's studies that are also in the same book are interesting too. He has separated a newborn dog from the other dogs, and after raising it for some time in a completely soft environment that would inflict no pain, he has shown that the dog did not recognize pain at first after it was put back into the normal environment. In a sense, this is a learned emotion. Pain is such a learned emotion that a pain from a burn and a pain from a knife stab are coded differently in the brain. Normally, they do not get mixed.

In my opinion, it is for this reason that it would be more effective to create suggestions according to the pain types of Ibn Sina.

If we turn to Erdine's book once again, we read that in reality, pain is not just a perceived experience but also an interpreted experience. Therefore, it differs from person to person. Factors such as the individual's personal and cultural characteristics, religion, gender and environment can change everything. Because in the end, a person perceives pain with his conscious, that means, his consciousness of pain develops.

Placebo, especially a placebo of an expensive drug could reduce pain. When a person is shot in the battlefield, he doesn't feel pain at that moment, until he reaches the hospital. The fear of death has covered the pain. And again, Erdine talks about the Big Bang Theory. According to the classical view, pain is a phenomenon that is perceived by the brain as passive. Because of these opinions that are based on the passive recording system, many pains have become incurable. But contemporary point of view says that a network consisting of the structures in the brain creates an ever-evolving internal reality that processes painful stimuli and other perceived data and memories.

According to the Big Bang Theory, six billion years ago, the evolution of the universe was determined within the first three minutes. Similarly, a long period of time is not always necessary for a pain to become chronical, long lasting. Pain can become chronic in a very short time. This experience is formed inside the memory. There, for this reason, Erdine says that the phrase, "An unpleasant feeling that benefits from all the past experiences of man," is included in the description of pain.

Unfortunately, although Erdine's book is a great work on pain and provides a complete description for it, hypnosis is mentioned with only a few sentences. Below is a short summary.

1. Pain is described by Ibn Sina, and different pains are coded in different ways in the brain.
2. Pain is a learned emotion.
3. Pain is an experienced and interpreted emotion.
4. The consciousness of pain develops differently in each person (Cultural, geographical)
5. Pain creates an internal reality in the brain.
6. Pain has a process that is formed in the memory and benefits from all the experiences of the past.
7. Pain is influenced when a different type of fear exists or when attention is focused on another point.

When we look at the seven items that form the pain mechanism, we can say that all seven factors in the mechanism can be addressed with hypnotherapy and that natural changes can be made...

We know that, with hypnotic suggestions, analgesia and anesthesia can be applied regionally or generally -other than dermatomes- and that a pain-free area at any region can be transferred to other places.

For instance, if we target the patient's hand and give the suggestion, "From now on, until my second suggestion, you will not feel pain or ache, or touching, burning, stinging sensations in the areas that I touch," we can remove pain in a marked area at the back of her hand. And to remove the pain-free region in the same subject, we say, "After this suggestion, you may feel pain or ache, or touching, burning, stinging sensations as before on the area at the back of your hand and at the places I had touched."

In order to transfer the pain-free area to another region, we say, "Now I am moving the pain-free area I have created at the back of your hand to the place I have marked on your abdominal region. As the back of your hand starts to feel pain again, now a pain-free area is being formed at the placed I have marked on your abdominal region."

The created pain-free areas can be conditioned with a keyword, and they can be recreated by saying the keyword without taking the subject under hypnosis.

HYPNOSIS AND ORGASM

Lack of vaginal pleasure

According to a survey, 40% of the women in Turkish society are unable to have vaginal pleasure. The causes for this are as follows.
1. Lack of sexual knowledge or experience
2. Fears of sexuality
3. Repulsion from sex
4. Lack of fantasies

Many women are able to have clitoral pleasure. They feel this kind of pleasure with touching or rubbing, and they may think that it is enough. The entrance of the penis and its penetration remains only mechanical. What they want is to perceive the touches of the penis at the clitoral area similarly at the vaginal area. When they cannot feel this, they enter a viscous cycle, in which they either accept the situation or act in order to please their partner. And some of them remain totally unresponsive.

The first three articles above may be overcome with education. Effective methods for lack of fantasies are the following.
1. Hypnodrama
2. Imagination
3. Creating physiological impact under hypnosis, simulation (Dr. Ulusoy)
4. Metaphors and stories

In order to apply the imagination method for lack of fantasy, it is important that the patient trusts her therapist. She has to be relaxed during suggestions for the treatment to be successful.

At this point, the therapist tries to expose her hidden dreams and fantasies.

It is as if she is being prepared for a sexual exploration journey. And hypnosis creates a *set/cover* effect for her to tell her therapist about the things that she is shy of about sexuality.

The therapist that will conduct sexual therapy must first be in peace with himself, he has to be able to remain neutral and not allow transference or counter-transference.

Hypnotherapy for Lack of Orgasm

Scientific studies have shown that orgasm is a mental condition. It is known that two hours of hypnotic exercises are enough to receive the orgasmic response from women who have previously experienced orgasm. But longer therapies are necessary for women who have never had an orgasm. (Dr. David Check)

We find the real or imagined reason of the problem with hypnoanalysis. In many of his studies, Dr. Check has found that the negative thoughts and perceptions learnt about love in early ages can create fear and guilt, thus preventing the women from having orgasms.

Dr. Check, who helped women relearn the approach to sex, also taught them under hypnosis that sex is a normal and fun activity, and not an activity that is evil and needs to be refrained from. While under hypnosis, the women thought about the fun parts of sexual activity and imagined touching their loved one with affection. They felt being touched at their genital region, being kissed and being touched all over their body. With the help of these exercises, the women were told how their body could experience sex and that sex was a good things.

Dr. Helen Singer Kaplan lists the stages of sex as follows.
1. Desire stage
2. Arousal stage
3. Orgasm stage

Desiring leads the person to interesting and passionate sexual activity.

Being aroused causes reactions in the body associated with sexual stimuli, and it creates physiological changes in the body with reflex mechanisms.

The orgasm stage is defined as the contraction -trembling- of reproductive organs.

If there is lack of vaginal fluid to ease penis penetration, or if there are spastic contractions at the vagina entrance that prevent penis entrance, we also talk about lack of sexual desire. But as an exception, many women, who have sexual desire and vaginal fluids, may also have vaginismus due to subconscious influences.

Many women to not feel pleasure during sexual intercourse. According to one of the prominent names in human sexuality research, Dr. H. Biegel, this insensitivity is not seen only during physical movement. But it is awakened singularly by sexual activity suggestions. Dr. Biegel used hypnosis to sensitize each of the organs that were previously insensitive. Through hypnosis, he made his patients relive the pleasure-giving feelings from the past (Feelings such as sucking, tickling, loving, caressing, bladder emptying or defecation, abdominal sensations while on a swing or sled, pleasant surprises, receiving an expensive present as a child, etc.). Then he used women's memories to provide sensitivity and pleasure to all their bodies, including the genital organs. By reliving these sensations, the women's feelings were aroused and they were once again able to have pleasure during sex.

It has been proven that, when a traumatic or disturbing event in the past merges with the negative thoughts about the event, it constitutes a cause for women's sexual problems. Hypnosis has an important role in displaying the devastating power of the event in the past, and also in the efforts to examine and remove the effects. (Dr. Richardson)

HYPNOTHERAPY FOR PREMATURE EJACULATION

The Method Applied to Couples – The Clay Vase Metaphor (Dr. Ulusoy)

Classically, blocking (Semans) and squeezing (Masters & Johnson) are reported to prolong the PE (Premature ejaculation) seen in man.

While anxiety is the primary factor in causing PE, it is possible to reduce anxiety and remove it with progressive relaxation exercises (PRT) and loosening techniques under hypnosis. A study has been conducted with two subjects; Sbj-1 was treated with hypnosis for his problem, and Sbj-2 was not in need of any treatment. When the relaxation level of Sbj-1 was compared to that of Sbj-2, it was seen that Sbj-1 had a more intensive relaxation but also that Sbj-2 had the same level of relaxation with the progressive relaxation technique.

The most important conclusion to be drawn is that, hypnotic relaxation can be used as a substitution for progressive relaxation. (Dr. Ulusoy)

I also think that prolonging the duration with blocking and squeezing in PE are not physiologically natural structures. (Dr. Ulusoy)

When the couple is taken into therapy for PE, as a representative system, a short film of an artist making a vase from clay (Mud) should be shown to the couple. The clay changes shape with each different touch and impact of the artist's fingers to the clay on the rotating disc. The couple is told that the intercourse they are going to have will be like making a vase out of clay. The clay is passive while the artist's fingers are active. The masterful touches of the fingers are almost like the flowing of the emotions in the mind to the clay. The clay prepares to change forms with those sweet, firm, sensitive touches. The couple is progressively taken into hypnosis.

To the male patient we say, "During sex, you are the artist who will make the clay vase... You have dreams, feelings, fantasies... You feel and experience the flow of your dreams, feelings and fantasies first to your hands...then to your fingers...and then to your penis that resembles your fingers..."

To the female patient we say, "You and your husband feel his fingers touch your body...the warmth, the sweet but firm touch of his penis at your wet and warm vagina... As your earthen body starts to take shape with your husband's sensual and penile touches, you feel yourself as an object being shaped..."

Then we turn to the man and say, "Yes, you feel your wife at your hands, your body, and at the most sensitive areas of your penis... From now on, your wife is an object to you, a piece of clay waiting to be shaped with your feelings and fantasies... Until you form the shape that you want from this clay, the most sensitive areas of your penis will remain the most insensitive..."

And then to the woman we say, "And you, the epitome of femininity, waiting to become a precious vase from clay... Until your husband gives you the shape he wants, continue to feel pleasure with your husband's touches with his finger and his penis as your desire and lust heighten... As you surrender all your earthen body to your husband, feel that you are being recreated with his every penile touch... You experience being reshaped... Feel his blows spreading from your stomach to your entire body..."

Then to the man we say, "Until all your fantasies are completed, until your desired shape is formed, the touches of your hands and the stiffness of your penis will continue..."

Then, in a way that they both can hear, we talk to the woman, "When you hear your husband say, 'The vase is almost finished' you will start panting and breathing rapidly, you will feel a pleasant vibration, a feeling of emptiness all over your body... When he says, 'It's done' you will feel small convulsions spreading from your stomach to your entire body..."

Related Videos:

http://www.youtube.com/watch?v=fzFBpy-LsQY

http://www.youtube.com/watch?v=4Jkipv08S34

DR. ULUSOY APPROACH TO ERECTILE DYSFUNCTION WITH HYPNOSIS

Erection problems are seen frequently. The reasons for disappointment could be due to the fact that the first experiences -especially in our society- occur in brothels with anxiety and hurry, and also because of the speedy ejaculations learned with masturbation, or because of lack of education, or of having the first experience on the first night of marriage. In addition, the stories man tell each other on penis diameter, size or duration records are also causes of anxiety.

In the training I provided at Üsküdar University on *Hypnotherapy in Sexual Problems*, I had cascaded my approach to sexual problems over seven steps.

Erectile dysfunction is a condition that is curable with hypnotherapy if morning stiffness exists. To patients with such problems, I apply the following process which is my personal approach.

1. Abreaction application for the event he has lived in the past which affects his current problem traumatically or atraumatically.
2. Providing relaxation suggestions.
3. Providing intercourse simulation suggestions.
4. Creating arm catalepsy, initiating non-hypnotic catalepsy with keyword, teaching how to continue and finish, providing the transfer of the cataleptic structure at the arm to the penis again with a keyword during intercourse.
5. Enabling rehearsal of the application in article four with intercourse simulation.
6. Creating hand anesthesia/insensitivity in order to prolong duration and to increase pleasure in future experiences, having the subject experience this and then carrying the senseless area at the hand to the penis tip with suggestion, building connection with a keyword group.
7. The keywords must be given double-sidedly such as, open - close or 0 - 1; meaning that there should be starting and ending commands.

The applications in items two and three decrease anxiety in the person. Anxiety is the leading actor in many sexual problems. Applications in articles four and five provide directly problem-oriented hypno-behaviorist conditioning. And the application in article six is used to prolong the duration in the future. A pain-free area can be created at the back of the hand and it can be tested with a needle, or senselessness may be provided with an iced-water simulation from an imaginary bucket.

In articles four and six, the mind is being provided with examples and then these examples are modelled. Because the mind is structured by building new models onto an information that it has learned with modelling.

DR. ULUSOY HYPNOSIS METHOD FOR ERECTION PROBLEMS AND PREMATURE EJACULATION – "KEYING"

We will be using two different methods together, both of which are hypnotic phenomena.

After the subject is taken under hypnosis, catalepsy is created on his right or left arm. To create catalepsy at the arm, we ask the subject to raise his arm parallel to the ground. While the arm is in the air, we hold his wrist with one hand. And with our other hand, we make a stroking motion from his shoulder to his fingertips. Before this motion, we say to the subject, "*I will be making a pass from your shoulder to your fingertips with my hand. All the areas my hand passes through will become stiff, hard as a wooden plank.*"

After the passing we make, the arm becomes stiff. We try to bend the arm but we cannot. We should make the subject experience the arm being unable to bend. Then we relax the arm with suggestions, saying, "*Now I will be making another pass from your shoulder to your arm. All the muscle groups that my hand passes over will become soft and loose, like cotton.*"

Then we need to give him a keyword to provide the stiffening and loosening of the arm.

"*Every time I say 'Four' your left arm will become stiff. Whenever I say 'Five,' it will loosen up and fall down. Now I want you to repeat my words after me, Every time I say 'Four' your left arm will become stiff. Whenever I say 'Five,' it will loosen up and fall down.*"

The subject will say, "Every time you say 'Four' my left arm will become stiff. Whenever you say 'Five,' it will loosen up and fall down."

Then we repeat, "*Every time I say 'Four' your left arm will become stiff. Whenever I say 'Five,' it will loosen up and fall down.*"

The subject is taken out of hypnosis and the keyword is checked. He puzzledly watches his left arm stiffen with the number four, and relax with the number five. Now he has control of his arm.

The subject is taken under hypnosis once again.

"*Now you have learned to control the stiffening and loosening at your arm with the keywords. I will transfer this model that you have learned to your penis for it to be filled with blood during intercourse and for it to become hard, stiff and to ejaculate and relax when the time comes.*

From now on, nothing will happen in your arm when I say four or five. I am transferring this model from your arm to your penis. When you repeat to yourself, 'Four, four, four' out of hypnosis, blood will fill into your penis and your penis will harden; when you say, 'Five, five, five' you will feel the stimulation at your penis tip intensively and as you ejaculate with this stimulus, the blood will return to your body from your penis, and your penis will slowly lose stiffness.

Now I want you to repeat after me, From now on, nothing will happen in your arm when I say four or five. I am transferring this model from your arm to your penis. When you repeat to yourself, 'Four, four, four' out of hypnosis, blood will fill into your penis and your penis will harden; when you say, 'Five, five, five' you will feel the stimulation at your penis tip intensively and as you ejaculate with this stimulus, the blood will return to your body from your penis, and your penis will slowly lose stiffness."

The subject will repeat, "From now on, nothing will happen in my arm when you say four or five. I am transferring this model from your arm to your penis. When I repeat to yourself, 'Four, four, four' out of hypnosis, blood will fill into my penis and my penis will harden; when I say, 'Five, five, five' I will feel the stimulation at my penis tip intensively and as I ejaculate with this stimulus, the blood will return to my body from your penis, and my penis will slowly lose stiffness."

Then we repeat, "*From now on, nothing will happen in your arm when I say four or five. I am transferring this model from your arm to your penis. When you repeat to yourself, 'Four, four, four' out of hypnosis, blood will fill into your penis and your penis will harden; when you say, 'Five, five, five' you will feel the stimulation at your penis tip intensively and as you ejaculate with this stimulus, the blood will return to your body from your penis, and your penis will slowly lose stiffness.*"

The subject is taken out of hypnosis. Stiffening and loosening have been created on the arm with keywords and this created model has been carried to the penis. The mind works with modelling. The subject is asked to use this keying during the first intercourse.

Also, at the beginning of this session, general body relaxation techniques are applied and the subject is given the suggestion that his mind and body will relax during intercourse. Because the main underlying reasons in many sexual problems, including erection, are stress and anxiety.

If the patient can become hard but has a premature ejaculation problem due to the sensitivity at his penis tip, similar modelling and keying may be done for this problem, too.

In such case, the above pattern is used. First, a pain-free area is created at the back of the hand, and a needle is stuck both under and out of hypnosis. Then, painlessness is coded with a keyword and the patient is asked to remove the pain with the keyword while out of hypnosis, and to stick himself with a needle. After taking out the needle, he is asked to remove the painlessness with the keyword.

Then, under hypnosis and with a suggestion that includes keywords, this model is taken from the back of the hand and it is transferred to the tip of the penis, which is highly sensitive and which triggers premature ejaculation. The patient is asked to desensitize the penis tip with the keyword right before he feels he will ejaculate.

CHAPTER 4

CLASSICAL TREATMENT IN VAGINISMUS AND VAGINISMUS DIARIES

This chapter is separate and independent of The Dr. Ulusoy Treatment Method. In this chapter classical treatment applications are mentioned and supported with vaginismus study diaries. It is aimed to take a look at the therapists who apply classical therapy, from the eye of the patient, and at the same time, it is aimed to help the patients, whom we define as simple vaginismus cases, to solve their problems with applications on their own. Moreover, a guideline is provided for patients applying to classical treatment to follow.

I would like to tell vaginismus patients about the story of the "Eagle's Flight of Rebirth" because stories make us think, they evolve and change us, guide us through life…

THE EAGLE'S FLIGHT OF REBIRTH

Flying to Freedom Once Again

Among bird species, eagles are the ones that live the longest. There are eagles that live up to seventy years. But in order to reach that age, it has to make a very serious and difficult decision while around the age of forty. When the eagle reaches the age of forty, its talons become hard and lose their elasticity, and therefore, the eagle becomes unable to grab on to the preys it needs to hunt for nutrition. Its beak becomes longer and bends toward its chest. Its feathers become tough and thick.

Now it has become really hard for the eagle to fly. So, the eagle has to choose from two options. Either it will choose death, or it will stand to the painful and formidable process of rebirth.

This rebirth process will last about 150 days. If it chooses this option, the eagle will fly to the top of a mountain and remain there on a rock wall, in its nest where it does not need to fly any more.

After finding such a convenient spot, the eagle starts banging its beak against the rock. In the end, the eagle's beak is torn off and it falls out. The eagle waits for its new beak to come out for a while. After his beak has grown out, he uses it to tear out its talons. And when the new talons come out, this time the eagle starts tearing off its old toughened feathers.

After five months, the eagle becomes ready to do the famous *flight of rebirth* that will bestow him with another twenty or so years of life.

VAGINISMUS EXERCISES

In classical vaginismus treatment, a process that lasts twelve weeks and that is carried out with weekly meetings is applied. During this process, training and finger exercises for the vagina penetration are provided. The main goal in finger exercises is to remove the contractions that are thought to originate from the lower 1/3 of vaginal muscles, and to enable the patient to experience the entry of something from the outside.

The classical definition of vaginismus contains the contraction of pelvic floor muscles. Therefore, the treatment plan suggests controlling the pelvic floor muscles.

This is the situation in the vaginismus cases we call secondary and that are mostly seen abroad. Couples, who have been having comfortable intercourse in the past, have this problem due to an existentialist or behaviorist trauma.

Therefore, finger exercises are given together with Kegel Exercises that are basically defined as "Holding and releasing as if you need to urinate."

But in the cases I have worked on since 2004, I have seen that in the vaginismus seen in Turks there are no problems at the lower 1/3 of vaginal muscles or at the pelvic floor muscles. And since there are no problems there, neither Kegel Exercises nor 12 weeks of finger exercises are relevant.

If you are able to understand the creation mechanism of a problem, you can easily provide the solution. As a cultural characteristic, the vaginismus seen in Turks is fear-based. This fear is manifested as panic attack symptoms, ranging from light to severe. Breathing turns into a rapid panting; the leg, back, upper back and neck muscles contract gradually. Withdrawal and pushing the partner away by hand are observed. All this originates from the mind, which has merged fear with a situation miscoded in the past while it was actually normal.

During the 2011 European Hypnosis Congress in Istanbul, I had revealed all of these differences in my vaginismus treatment studies from 450 cases.

In the treatment that will be an alternative for classical treatment, the aim is to remove the contractions observed in the outer body, and to provide mind-body harmony, triple feedback exercises (Can something go inside? Can the increase in diameter be tolerated? Are there any problems with the hymen?), and suggestion - breathing control exercises are utilized.

Exercises for vaginismus treatment exist also in our treatment method but still, they are less in number and only aimed at receiving answers on whether something can go inside, can the increase in diameter be tolerated, and whether there are any problems with the hymen. Because in the vaginismus seen in Turks, the lower vaginal muscles and the pelvic floor muscles are loose.

When you look at the problem from the correct point of view, which means being problem-oriented, then the solution can come in an average of *one and a half days* within three phases. This is why we call our treatment *The Three-Phase Method.*

In this section, firstly the classical treatment will be explained and the *exercise and success experiences* of two patients, who were classically treated, will be conveyed via their diaries. In addition, examples will be provided from of treatment processes from the 146 patients, who were classically treated and who succeeded with the free of charge support I provided for one year in a Yahoo group during 2005 and 2006.

At the same time, this section where the classical treatment is explained will be guiding for therapists and it will also include application patterns for patients with simple vaginismus who don't have the chance to receive treatment.

HYMENS

Hymens may show a lot of variety. They may be ring, half-moon or double-ring shaped, thin, veined, veinless, elastic or hard.

The hymens of Turkish women are mostly elastic and either half-moon or ring shaped.   We see these types of hymens in every four out of ten women we work with. While these hymens allow penetration, they don't bleed either. They are mostly deformed during childbirth.

One of the false myths of Turkish women is the hymen being ruptured. Saying that it will be deformed rather than ruptured is a softer way of expressing it. The belief of rupturing is so intense that the woman thinks that she will feel pain with cognitive distortions like explosion, extensive bleeding, the blood splattering around and on the walls, that her eyes will pop out, or that something like a broomstick or a leg of a table will be entering.

All of these are false beliefs, which we call myths and which are spread on the grapevine. Such false beliefs, together with many other factors, are also the causes of vaginismus.

First of all, our youngsters should know that the hymen is nothing to be afraid of. And it is also important for men to know that not every hymen will bleed so that they will not have any arguments about virginity.

Unfortunately, in some cases, in which the women had serious contractions and in which we completed treatments with great hardship, there have been men who left their wives shortly after the first experience because there was no bleeding. For this reason, at the beginning of my treatment, I make sure to give information about hymens. If there is no bleeding during the exercises or during the experience, I remind them that four out of ten hymens are elastic. Nevertheless, if I still some doubt in the man, I put the related literature in front of him and make him read them. But in some cases the man sees his wife's severe contractions, he knows that she could not have had sex with such contractions, and despite all the information I provide him with, he still falls in doubt and divorces his wife after treatment.

And then there are cases that exemplify the saying, "God works in mysterious ways!" There has been a time when a man, who had divorced his wife because he thought that she was not a virgin, came back to us with his second wife due to vaginismus. And he experienced that his second wife also had an elastic hymen and that she did not bleed.

Rarely, if the hymen is problematic, it can be surgically operated.

Where is the hymen? Most of the women think that the hymen is deep inside the vagina but in fact, the hymen is at the entrance of the vagina, at the point where you can feel the vagina entrance with one node of your finger.

For pictures on hymen types, please check the "Pictorial Representation" section below.

VAGINISMUS FINGER EXERCISES

"In classical treatment"

Generally three main factors are important in vaginismus treatment.
1. Education
2. Removal of contractions with hypnotherapy (In cases where hypnotherapy is not used, physical muscle stretching and loosening exercises, as well as finger exercises are given as homework in order to remove contractions, as in classical treatment. Homeworks are behaviorist treatments and they aim to control the mind via the vagina, and to control the body -the muscle groups- via the mind. *Whereas in hypnotherapy, by directly interfering with the mind, it is possible to replace the contractions in the body with relaxation, to ensure that the homeworks are done easily, and to enable the patient to be examined comfortably when necessary.*)
3. Vaginal exercises for checking whether something can go in, or whether there is a problem with the diameter increase or with the hymen

Some of the patients are not happy with the homework on the vagina and they don't want to do them. According to the triple model above, exercises are necessary for a good treatment. There are also situations in which the contractions are removed with hypnotherapy and where the intercourse is experienced. But the homework being completed, the patient recognizing, feeling her genital region, and the patient experiencing the expandability of her vagina are important in terms of her transferring the authority to her husband, and they also ease the initiation of intercourse.

Pictorial Representation

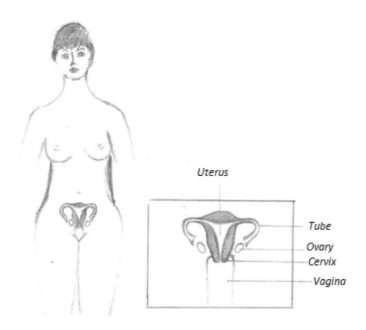

Pic-1: Taken from the book *Completely Overcome Vaginismus*, modified and redrawn by A. Ayşe Yalçındağ

The organ that we call uterus extends toward the ovaries with tubes left and right. And at the bottom, it droops to the vagina. Below, the vagina reaches the outside through an opening called hymen that is between the inner lips. The vagina is four to five inches on average. With this condition, a woman's internal genital structure is located at the lower abdominal cavity.

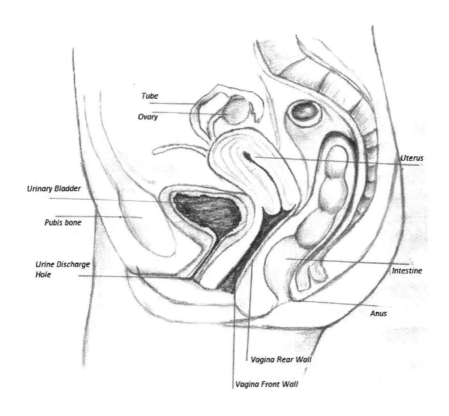

Pic-2: Taken from the book *Completely Overcome Vaginismus,* modified and redrawn by A. Ayşe Yalçındağ

When we look from the side, from the front to the back we see the joining point of the pubis bone, behind it is the urinary bladder, vagina front wall, vagina rear wall, intestines and the anus exit. Normally, the front and rear vagina walls stand on top of each other. When something goes in, depending on the diameter of the entering object, they open up like a sock to surround it. Normally they open around 2.9 inches, and they open up to 4.3 inches at child delivery with the effect of hormones. And an approximately 1.4 inch opening is enough for the penis to enter.

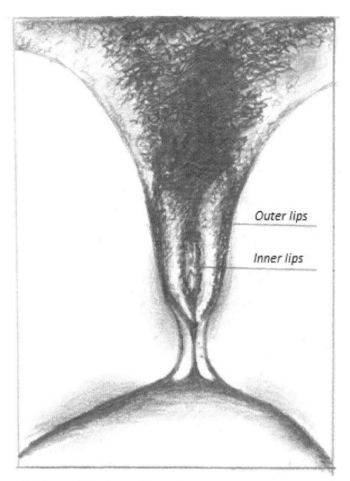

Pic-3: Taken from the book *Completely Overcome Vaginismus*, modified and redrawn by A. Ayşe Yalçındağ

When we look from the outside, we see the outer lips and the inner lips inside them.

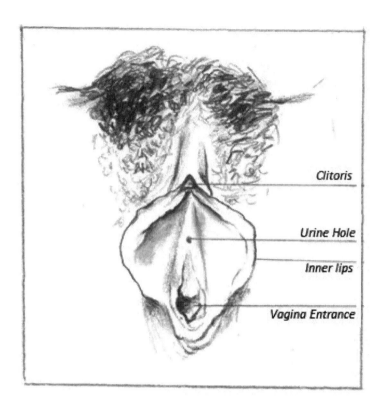

Pic-4: Taken from the book *Completely Overcome Vaginismus,* modified and redrawn by A. Ayşe Yalçındağ

The vaginismus patient should especially get to know her genitalia by help of a mirror. When she looks from the outside, she sees the outer and inner lips. When she parts the outer and inner lips, at the top joining point of the inner lips, she will see the pleasure organ, which we call the *clitoris,* the female equivalent of the penis in man. There is the urinary hole in the middle, and the vaginal opening at the bottom. The vaginal opening is not a general opening as seen in the pictures. It seems to be closed because of the vaginal walls standing on top of each other.

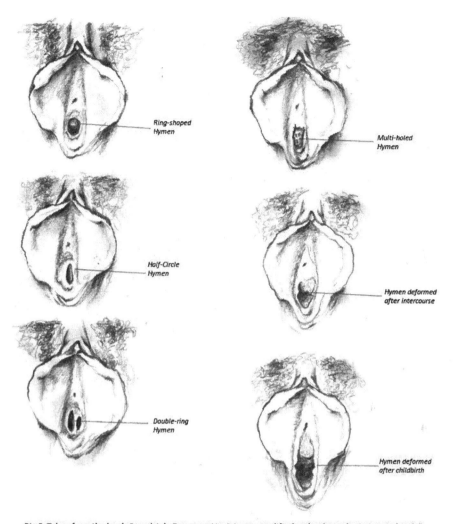

Labels in figure: Ring-shaped Hymen; Multi-holed Hymen; Half-Circle Hymen; Hymen deformed after intercourse; Double-ring Hymen; Hymen deformed after childbirth

Pic-5: Taken from the book *Completely Overcome Vaginismus*, modified and redrawn by A. Ayşe Yalçındağ

Hymens seen as ring, half-ring and double-ring shaped, multi-holed, deformed after intercourse and deformed after childbirth.

Our patient's first homework should be about looking, seeing, touching and feeling the vagina entrance. Each finger exercise needs to be done ten to twenty times a day until the next session.

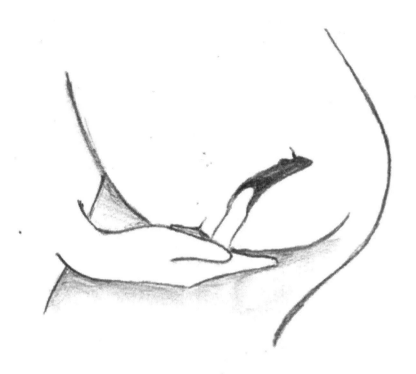

Pic-6: Taken from the book *Completely Overcome*
Vaginismus, **modified and redrawn by A. Ayşe Yalçındağ**

The second homework involves the patient placing her finger at the vagina entrance that she has felt earlier, and breathing correctly to lead the finger inside. (Correct breathing is described at the end of the book, under the title *Breathing.*) One finger goes in one node first, then two nodes and then three nodes. In classical treatments, this exercise is spread over three weeks.

After the first homework, our patient has experienced the fact that something can go inside. The following homework is structured on the increasing of the diameter, rather than something going inside.

In the third homework, two fingers (Index and middle fingers) are taken inside, one node first, then two nodes and then three nodes. In classical treatments, this exercise is also spread over three weeks.

The fourth homework is taking in one finger of the partner and then two fingers. In this exercise, the authority is passed on to the partner. Before the experience, the partner's finger provides the intermediation and acceptance before the penis.

In classical treatments, intercourse is not advised before the exercises are completed. The main rule is for the couples to recognize, touch and feel each other's bodies, and for the exercise to be completed.

In The Dr. Ulusoy Method, vaginal exercises are used short-term for receiving the following feedback.
1. Can something go in?
2. Can she tolerate the increase in diameter?
3. Is there a problem with the hymen?

In The Doctor Ulusoy Method, after the finger exercises and all other exercises are completed within the same day, taking in the partner's finger is also done for a short period and the transfer of authority is thus provided.

The significant difference of The Dr. Ulusoy Method with the classical treatment is that it allows all the exercises to be completed with three meetings/phases within the same day that the patient comes in for treatment by,
1. Removing contractions and providing relaxation with hypnosis,
2. Providing homework doability with suggestions.

After gradual problem-oriented hypnotherapy, our patient becomes able to do the vaginal exercises she is given. If there are any patients, who are unable, who are stuck at any phase (15%), solution is reached after a short-term simple examination and exercise, because she has already had hypnotherapy earlier. Having had hypnotherapy also makes it easy to work on patients who have fear of being medically examined. Primary emphasis is especially put on controlling the hip, breathing and legs.

VAGINISMUS DIARIES

This section is especially meant for patients. It has been designed for those who are unable to seek treatment due to financial reasons. *Vaginismus Diary 1* includes all the homework practices, and more importantly, all the details of the experiences during the practices of a vaginismus patient who has had classical treatment for twelve weeks with weekly meetings. As you will see below, this vaginismus patient has noted all the homework and practices to the finest detail.

The following *Vaginismus Diary 2* has revised the given homework and practices according to her personality structure, rendering them more compatible with her.

As can be seen in the diaries and as I had especially mentioned in my vaginismus classification, personality structures are also important in vaginismus treatment.

"While thinking about presenting you the vaginismus finger exercises work schedule, I found it more appropriate to give you the homework practices of Ayşe and Deniz (Both are nicknames). Because Ayşe and Deniz are similar to you, they have carried out the exercises and personally experienced the difficulties just like you..."

VAGINISMUS DIARY 1

Dear Friends,

Firstly, it is best that you have yourself examined by a physician to be definitely diagnosed with vaginismus. Because sometimes the person can self-diagnose herself as vaginismus but the problem may actually be physical, such as a structural anomaly, endometriosis disease, etc. This why an examination by a physician is an absolute must.

Another thing I want to prioritize is the fact that you should push your means and get help from a professional that determines your treatment process specifically for you. The things I am writing here are for those who do not have the means to see a physician and who are only looking for things they can do on their own. But I also need to say that the physicians who apply the behaviorist approach will tell you the same things, more or less. Therefore, ask the physician what kind of therapy he will be using. You already receive the behaviorist approach and motivation from the website and the group. As you know, the number of women who have overcome their problem with the strength they got from the website is quite many...

As the causes of the vaginismus problems are psychological -inner world oriented- the years that pass by without intervention cause the situation to be cast in cement... But if you haven't really received a serious therapy, you are not late at all... I believe this is what you need to be thinking first; do you believe that you can overcome your vaginismus by getting used the feeling that something go into that area? If your problem is limited to this, we can overcome it...

You need to determine at which level your sexual relationship is. Is there everything other than vaginal intercourse? Or is there also frigidity, the removal of sex from your marriage? This is important.

I received therapy at the sexual dysfunction unit of a private hospital for about three months. Since our only problem was fear of the penis, sexual intimacy (Foreplay, etc.) was not forbidden. In some vaginismus therapies, physicians forbid sexual intimacy too. This is good for some couples but it harms others. Because if you take sex out of your life completely, you are also hindering your sexual impulses and pleasure while trying to solve your vaginismus. But on the other side, applying a sex diet relieves the patient from that pressure for a while and helps her to be relaxed while making love because she thinks that there won't be intercourse at the end. I think you should make the distinction this way; if you have really become alienated from sex and if you don't even want to make love to your husband, don't have any sexual intimacy while doing these exercises. Never try sexual relationship while doing these eleven-stage exercises or you will have to return to the beginning. (What I mean by sexual relationship here is not about taking out kissing, caressing, etc. out of your life; it only means to refrain from touching the genital areas.) In short, there should be no trials of penetration to the genital area by hand or with the penis. Sometimes, with the progress you make, you may fall into momentary carelessness by thinking that you are doing well and that maybe a trial with the penis could be done. But don't. The result will be disappointment, causing you to start the exercises all the way from the beginning, and all your previous efforts will go to waste. We are not in a hurry; if we have waited for so long, we can wait another three months, right? (In any case, I would like to remind you that the duration can become longer or shorter, depending on the person.)

Before starting the exercises, it would be greatly helpful if you examine the female anatomy from a good source. It is always good to embark on an expedition by studying the map first. Learn well about the locations and features of the vagina, genital area, uterus, ovary, etc. from the internet or books. Do research on what happens during intercourse, how far does the penis enter, what kind of chemical changes occur at the vagina and the rest of the body, etc. Sometimes lack of a very simple knowledge could cause vaginismus. And sometimes, a piece of information that you never knew before could help you in your journey.

The vagina is like the palm of a newborn baby; whatever you put inside, it will take that object's shape. As it is a completely muscular structure, it takes shape according to the size and shape of the incoming object. Vaginismus is not the contraction of the entire vagina, as most of us would think. It is only the contraction at the first inch or so at the entrance[7]. So in fact, the enemy is much simpler than the one we create in our heads. But yet, the "Contract!" instruction coming from the brain is so strong that the whole area becomes almost like a wall; it becomes fully stiff. Our aim here is to practice determination, patience and discipline in order to teach the brain that it will not feel pain. In this sense, I am going to write down in detail about everything that you need to do step-by-step. May it be easy for you. Believing is halfway to success; I believe that you will succeed. Love…

Now, step-by-step, I am writing the stages of the exercises that you need to do.

First, get yourself a notebook. You will write down your exercises daily. (This will increase your courage as you see the stages you have passed, and it will also measure where you are at in your therapy. So you will see how much you are ready to pass to the upper stage.)

The following information will be recorded on each page of the notebook.
1. The date you did the exercise
2. The finger you used during the exercise
3. How many trials you had
4. Contraction value. Here, you will assign a self-determined value, from zero to ten. For instance, when you are extremely contracting, you can give it ten, and when you don't contract at all, you can give it zero. Evaluate the contraction as the pain you feel. (Please make sure to apply the same criteria for the score you give for the contraction intensity because the measurement and the decision to pass to the next stage will be made by taking these values as basis.)
5. The total duration of your daily exercises. (This duration should be at least

---

(7) **Author's note**: As Ayşe has been treated by a classical therapist, she thinks that the problem comes from the contracting of the lower vagina muscles. But as I have seen in my studies and experiences, and as I have presented at the congresses, the vagina is loose in the vaginismus of Turkish women. The real problem is the panic, fear, wholebody contractions, withdrawal and the irregularity in breathing.

half an hour. As you increase the duration, the reinforcement will also be increased, so the solution will come quicker.)

This is how you can understand if you are doing the scoring correctly or not.

"As the score of your contractions goes down, the number of entries should increase. As the number of entries increase, your contraction score should decrease."

Here is an example for the notes you need to take:

Date	Which finger – How many nodes	Number of entries	Contraction Value (1-10)	Duration (Mins.)
March 1	Pinky finger - 1 node	10	7	30

Exercises:

Before starting the exercises, I want to give you some advice; if you agree, just read the explanation of the stage that you are currently in. Do you want to know why? First of all, it is more exciting to pass each stage and to wonder about the next one, and also, it could be better not to read the latest stages that could make you feel that you can't do them. I am not saying this because the steps you will take are difficult. What I'm trying to say is something like entering a contest and knowing what all the questions are. Would you still feel like solving them? But it is your choice. May it be easy for you; I wish you success.

1. **First Stage**: With the palm of your hand and sometimes with your fingers, apply some pressure and touches onto that region (Outer genital, outer and inner lips). The goal is to get that region accustomed to touching and feeling. At least half an hour every evening. By the way, here is a question for you: Have you ever stood in front of a mirror and examined that region? No? Do this immediately. (I had done even the first stages of the finger exercises in front of the mirror; it was very effective in providing motivation!)

2. **Second Stage**: With any of your fingers that you feel comfortable with, try a single node entry. If you look at your finger from the pam side, you will see two lines. These lines divide the finger into three equal pieces, and each of these pieces is a node. You will try entry up to the first node line. Take a deep

breath first. Assume a sitting position that feels comfortable. You should not have any clothes at the lower part. You can get one of the water-based gels (OK or Durex) that are sold in pharmacies. They are perfect products that provide lubricity during exercises. In fact, as you do the exercises you will also notice that there is no pain when there is lubricity. If you cannot buy a gel, you can also use the familiar baby oil[8]. But still, I advise these gels more because there is a lot of difference between the two. By the way, it is very important for your fingernails to be short-cropped and clean so that you don't get an infection. Your nails should also be free of scratching unevenness, which we call hangnails...

Take a deep breath. Use the gel to wet your finger (The parts that will enter)... And slowly push this first node inside... Don't hurry and fall into dishearten-ment... In my first trials, I was saying, "No, it won't happen. No way it can go in there." But in later stages, I took in two fingers and then the penis... The trick here is to go step by step. You pushed your finger in and saw that you have intensive contractions. Stop and wait, for half an hour if needed. Just wait like that, until is passes... Early on, I used to wait for twenty to thirty minutes for one entry until the contraction went away. You would not believe me but I used to just wait there in front of the TV... Find something to pass time; read a book or watch TV... But if there is no contraction, there is no waiting... If you are able to allocate the time, increase the duration of the exercise from half an hour to one hour, even more... Because the exercise intensity in the early stages is important. After making the finger entrance, if there is no contrac-tion, take it out and try again without waiting. This way, take the notes I have described above on how many entries you made in half an hour, what was the value of your contraction, etc. You will do these for one week.

Never lose hope; I have been through the same path. There were times when I said, "This won't happen with the finger. No, I can't. I'll quit," but I didn't give up. You should not give up either. Nothing is impossible in life.

By the way, you might ask which position you need to be in. You know the examination couches of gynecologists, the ones that scare us (Especially us vaginismus women) even while looking at them. There, the position assumed at that couch is the ideal position for the vagina to be raised and to open fully. But when you try the exercises in this position, you need to lay down on your back and lift your legs slightly. It will also help easy penetration if you spread your legs too. Another detail: I had had great difficulty while doing the first node and I could not get my finger inside no matter what position I took. At one point, I remember trying this and it had really helped: After taking off

---

(8)   **Author's Note:** We don't advise baby oil because it is oil-based.

your under clothes, squat down and try it that way. (It could hurt less when stretched.) It could be different for each person but it worked for me. I had tried it this way in the first few days.

By the way, another important point about the exercises is that, if you push the vagina outwards as you do while defecating[9], the opening at the entrance will increase and make entries easier. In the first days that you start doing the exercises, your finger, your hand, arm or shoulder could become stiffened. And this is normal. Don't fall into despair. This is nothing more than your brain realizing an entry trial to that region and diverting the familiar "Contract!" command to other places. In fact this is a positive development because the vagina is moving the contraction feeling away from that region by transferring it to other organs. (But don't worry if your shoulder doesn't become stiff while exercising; don't make me regret saying this! ☺) The contractions in that region will pass in time; keep up the exercises…

Also, there is an exercise that enables you to control the muscles in that region. Try to do this every time you can during the day. I am talking about Kegel Exercise[10]. There were detailed explanations about it on the website. You can look there to see how it is done. This exercise is not just good for helping you control the muscles in that region, but it also provides you to get more pleasure from sex after you overcome vaginismus. It has another benefit: It helps you to recover from the looseness that occurs at the vagina after child delivery, and also helps you to return to active sex life quicker.

You need to continue this second stage three or four nights a week (Every night if you have the time; that was what I did), for at least half-hour periods. Don't forget that this initial stage of finger exercises is the week where you need to motivate yourself the most, when you need to be strongest. Don't tell me that you cannot spare the time; forget about evening gatherings, visits, etc. for a while. As in every job, this also needs strict pursuance and concentration. Don't ever skip this half-hour exercises in the evenings. As the most important thing in your life is to get rid of this problem, it is very important that you make this sacrifice. If you continue with discipline and patience, I am sure you will overcome your vaginismus in a period of three months. In the meanwhile, your husband's support is very important, too. It is important that he is by your side while you do the exercises, that he holds your hand when you are frustrated

---

(9)   **Author's Note:** Taking in while pushing out is a wrong application.

(10) **Author's Note:** As the ethiology of the vaginismus seen in Turks is different, Kegel Exercises are not relevant. The vagina is loose in Turkish women.

and want to give up, that he makes sure you don't let go, and that he puts aside the friendly visits for a while and motivates you to do the exercises.

During this first week of finger exercises, you did the one finger, one node entries at least four nights and wrote down your notes regularly. Take a look at your notes; how many entries have you tried on average per half hours, what is your average contraction score? Here, the main point is how comfortable you feel about moving on to the next stage. When you evaluate yourself and look at your notes to see how you have progressed, are you able to say, "Yes, I can move on to the next stage"? If the answer is "Yes," you may now go on to the next stage. Here, as an example, I will present in the appendix what my scores were when moving to the next stage. (But if I need to give a rough figure just for you to have an idea about it, in the half-hour exercises done at least three times a week, if you are able to record eighty entries and two or less contraction value, it will be enough for you to move on to the next stage. Here, we talk about three consecutive days because sometimes a comfortable exercise day may be specific to that certain day, so a minimum three-day period of enhancement is required.)

Important: Continuing each step for at least one week will ensure that you move along the steps saturatedly so it will make it more easy and comfortable for you to move to further steps, and it will also help you be much more comfortable at the final penis stage.

3.   **Third Stage**: You have passed the first step of finger exercises and now you are the one finger, two nodes level. First of all, I must tell you that you have pulled through the most difficult part. Because now that you have come aboard the ship to embark on the journey, you can believe in yourself from now on. It will not be long before you reach the opposite shore. This stage is simpler and the rule is exactly the same. Push it in, stop if you have contractions, wait until they go away, once they do, take it out and repeat without pause. Having burning sensations, contractions, repulsions, feeling out whatever is inside and after all these, feeling doubt whether your vagina is normal or not... All this is normal. You are healing. Take your notes again. If you are comfortable at this stage and if you are able to go through three consecutive days comfortably -with low contraction scores- pass on to the next stage.

4.   **Forth Stage**: We are at the last step of the exercises that you will do with one finger. One finger, three nodes. The most common mistake at this stage is going on an exploration trip on your vagina like a gynecologist. Don't forget, there is no exploration, no acting as a gynecologist. We will just learn how not to feel pain. Otherwise, if you take that trip, your attention will be

distracted toward other places with obsessions on whether you are normal or if your vagina is normal.

By the way, as your progress into the vagina has become longer, I advise you to apply some of the gel to your vagina. The gel on your finger may not be enough.

5.   **Fifth Stage (Double finger stages)**: This stage is a milestone, just as the one finger, one node step was. Because this is the step that you will find most difficult but also the one that is closest to success. Therefore, it is very important that you arrive at this stage after passing the previous steps very very comfortably. At this stage, your husband also joins in the exercises. So his support, his accompaniment is very important. Now, this part of our exercise consists of two levels.

i.   The level with your two fingers and one node
ii.   The level with your husband's one finger and one node

You will do the first half hour by yourself and the second half hour with your husband. It is important that the exercise with your husband is right after your solo exercise. So, don't work with your husband's finger first. The order is important. This way, it will be easier to take one finger of your husband after taking in two of your own fingers, and you will be taking the first step toward taking in a foreign object.

Join two fingers (Index and middle fingers) at the tips. Wet them with gel. Then take them in as in the previous exercises. Again, the rule is the same, "Push it in, stop if you have contractions, wait until they go away, and repeat without pause." Here, there are a few things you need to pay attention to; don't take in one finger, then the other. You need to take both of them in at the same time. Because the main objective here is not to stuff the fingers inside in any way possible, but to make the brain accept and adapt to the difference in thickness at the entrance. What we are trying to make the brain adapt to is, "First the thickness was less, I taught you how not to feel pain. Now I am giving you something thicker, you will learn how to take in without pain, too." So try to take both fingers in at one go. It is normal for you to have difficulty or contractions while taking in two fingers and one node because slowly, you are arriving at the penis size. It is really very normal for your brain to send the "Contract!" signal. Never give up. Don't forget, we cannot give in to this enemy that is only an inch long. Success is near; please keep your inner strength high. We all went through these phases. You too, have the right to be a healthy woman, to become a mother.

You have completed the part of the exercises that were only about you, and you took your notes. It is very normal for the number of your entries to go down, for your contractions to increase. Don't be upset; everything is going to get better.

Now it is time for the phase with your husband. It is important that your husband's hands are clean and his fingernails are short. Just as you did, he too, will put gel on his finger and do entry trials just like you did. There is something important here; your husband's finger should be under your control. In fact, you should be the one to push and pull the finger; this is necessary for the first steps. It gives you confidence. You are taking in an object, other than your body, inside for the first time; it is very important that you feel confident. At this point, some husbands may want to make jokes by moving their finger while inside. Don't let them do that because the slightest movement could make you think that you have lost control and you may get scared. It is important that you are in total control during the first steps. What have we done? We put gel on your husband's finger and we pushed it in slowly. It could be just one node or even just a small piece, just as much as you feel comfortable. We are not in a hurry. We are waiting, naturally we are having contractions, wait, wait… until the contraction goes away. When it is gone, pull the finger out quickly and then push it back in without pausing. At the point when you believe that you are comfortable during the exercises done with your husband, let him take control. Until then, you will have become accustomed to a penetration by something other than yourself. And now that your husband has joined in the exercises, you two have become a tight team that gives each other determination, strength and that are always there for each other. Had you ever been so close to each other? Think about all the other things you and your husband will overcome in this marriage together… ☺

It is important not to pass on to the second node before feeling comfortable at this stage. Because the thickness that you are experiencing has increased, and also, you are in contact with a foreign object other than your body, for the first time. On the scores that you put down in your notebook, if the scores for your solo exercises are enough to pass on to the next stage but the scores of the exercises with your husband's finger are not enough, or vice versa, then you will continue until the scores are close. (If the average number of entries is around eighty per half-hour and if your average contraction value is under two -naturally the reduction of contraction values will be parallel to an increase in entry trials- then you can go on to the next stage.) That was how it had happened with me. Although I was more relaxed with my husband's finger, I was having a hard time with my own fingers. So we kept on working during the following week until our values got closer.

Again, to see the details of my diary at this stage and in the two-finger exercises, check the table at the end.

6.   **Sixth Stage**: Have you been able to go through the steps of the previous stage with your two fingers and with your husband's finger? Do your scores match the criteria we have set for passing on to the upper stage? Can you say, "I can take my husband's finger, and one node of my own two fingers easily. I do not have contractions and my entry numbers have increased"? Then now you can move on to the exercises with your two fingers, two nodes and with your husband's one finger, two nodes. The rule is the same; work half an hour solo, half an hour with your husband. (One after the other; don't forget that enhancement is key!) If there is a lot of difference between the scores of your solo work and that of your collective work, repeat the same exercise the following week.

Caution: We don't use three nodes in the exercises you do with your own two fingers.

7.   **Seventh Stage**: Now you are easily able to take in two of your fingers to two nodes, and one of your husband's fingers to one node. At this stage of the exercises, we leave out your fingers and continue working with your husband's finger. Since you have worked with one node of your husband's finger in the previous stage, now we will have it easy. At this stage, we will work with your husband's one finger and two nodes.

8.   **Eighth Stage**: We will work with your husband's one finger and three nodes. Our general rules always remain the same, of course.

9.   **Ninth Stage**: After successfully managing three nodes with your husband's finger, now it is time for the exercises you will do with your husband's two fingers. The same rules as in the work with our own two fingers also apply here. The only difference is that the two fingers going in don't belong to us. But we are already familiar with our husband's finger from the previous stage, so I don't think you will have any problems. But as the thickness has changed, you just need a little bit more effort. Let your husband join two fingers at the tips. Apply plenty of gel and push in while you are in total control of the fingers. What was our rule? Push in, wait if you contract, when it is over pull them back and then repeat. (Hang on, it's almost over!)

10.   **Tenth Stage**: The entry trials with your husband's two fingers and two nodes.

11. **Eleventh Stage**: The entry trials with your husband's two fingers and three nodes.

Important: Don't move on to the upper stage before you see that you are truly comfortable with the previous one, because you are very close to the final. These lower stages are the infrastructure works for the performance you will display at the final. (By the way, use more of the gel during the stages with your husband. Being wet will relax the vagina.)

12. **Penis Stage**

12.1 **One node stage with the penis**: Now it is time for the exercises you will do with the penis. ☺

I had had the most difficulty with the two-finger stage. After that, the penis stage felt easy to me because the finger is rough, like a rod and it is more difficult for the vagina to take its shape when compared to the penis. Whereas the penis is built for the vagina, so its ergonomics is much more suitable for the vagina. That was why I had had a great surprise with the penis. At this stage, you will take in only the tip (Up to the point where the ringed area ends) of the penis. We suggest the position in which you are on top. Apply plenty of gel to the tip of the penis and into the vagina. (It is very important that you are adequately wet here.) And again the same rule; push, wait in case of contraction, pull back when it's gone, then again without waiting. Think of the penis just like a finger, you are not at the point of intercourse yet. At this point of the exercise, spouses (Especially men) may not be able to hold themselves back and try to go further. And that is one of the greatest mistakes you could make. Don't ever go any further, just the tip. Don't forget. Don't do it even if you are the one who wants it. At least not while at the penis tip step. Impatience at this step might require you to go back a few steps in your exercises. So, no hurry, no breaking the rules. If we lose discipline, we may have to start from the beginning... You may have this problem at this stage of the exercises: Your husband might have problems staying erect. And at this point, as doing this exercise depends on your husband standing erect, it is very important for him to be psychologically comfortable and persevering. So don't put any pressure on yourself or on your husband. Let it be as much as possible. It may not be easy to keep notes at this stage so don't pester yourself; you can give approximate values. In this section of the exercise, you may suddenly feel yourself stuck in the middle of a struggle between your husband's erection and you vagina. Like I said; relax. No hurries. Liven up the exercise with foreplay, etc. to help with his erection.

12.2 **Two nodes stage with the penis**: Don't forget that it will be very helpful to apply plenty of gel to the penis and vagina before the exercise.

12.3 **The entire penis stage**: And now, all of the penis... Now your entries must have become much easier. Using plenty of gel is necessary to provide adequate wetness during the penis stages. At this step, it is important to work intensively enough to increase the number of penetrations. This way, you will slowly arrive to the point of practicing the in and out motions of real intercourse.

I assume you have been able to take in the entire penis in one of these last weeks. Now I will offer you some positions for easier entries. At the first entry, you had done it while you were on top. If that beginning is ideal for you, continue that way until you are totally comfortable. The position with you on top gives you complete control so it makes you better taste the feeling of confidence. And you can arrange the entrance depth of the penis more easily in this position. But sometimes, having the control to yourself may not be enough for the depth. In fact, that was what had happened with me; while I was on top, we could only move to half of the first node and afterwards I could not go any further, as if the road had ended. At this point, the position below came in very handy.

Sit at the edge of the bed with your legs toward the floor and your back leaning on the bed. (A pillow under your lower back would be helpful by raising you up.) You husband will be standing. After applying plenty of gel into the vagina, hold the penis and try to take it in slowly while you have full control of it, as if it was a finger. Go as much as you can and stop when you feel pain. Don't go any further. Just wait in that position, just as in the finger exercises. When the contraction goes away, take it out and push it back in. Try it this way for a while. Yes, you may have difficulty at first but it will become easier as you try. Everything will get better. Before your intercourses, try with your two fingers and gel as practice. This will be comforting during the first times. And you will see that you will discover new methods as you try, and you will become more comfortable in time. Burning sensations, the need to urinate (Because the vagina is neighbors with the urinary bladder), feeling of pressure, etc. are all normal. The vagina is trying to get used to a full intercourse for the first time with the in and out motions. So, everything you are going through is completely normal; give yourself some time. Even for a woman who doesn't have vaginismus, getting used to sexuality, noticing and feeling the different types of touches at the vagina, and her discoveries on the path to pleasure could take up to one or one and a half years on average. So just give yourself time; everything will get better in time. Explore each other with your spouse. Everything will be better with the efforts. Always have love in your hearts and happiness in your home...

(Don't forget to say a prayer, okay?) Love...

Nickname: Ayşe Koşlu

TABLES OF EXERCISE DIARIES

Day 1

Finger	Depth	Entries	Contraction (0-10)	Duration	
Index	Half a node	13	6	30 min.	*As you can see, I wasn't able to take in a single node in the first days.*

My feelings: When I take my finger in, I get the reflex to push it out like a finger in my throat. It doesn't keep the finger inside, it slowly loosens up and lets it go. High level of pushing the finger out. I've given up already. God, give me strength.

Day 2

I wasn't feeling well, I couldn't try at all... — *This was a lie. I was trying to escape, slowly giving up, making up excuses.*

Day 3

Finger	Depth	Entries	Contraction (0-10)	Duration	
Index	4 half, 3 full nodes	7	6	15 min.	*It becomes difficult when you skip a day. The most important factor in the exercises is the principle of enhancement.*

My feelings: Is the path really straight forward after the vagina entrance? It feels like there is a cartilage-like bump at first... I feel terribly nauseous while taking the finger out There is a bump at the entrance, the path is not flat. I feel nauseous even while touching the area outside of the vagina. I am terribly nauseous. The vagina is pushing the finger back out.

Day 4

Finger	Depth	Entries	Contraction (0-10)	Duration	
Index, Middle	1 node	6	7	20 min.	*It was like torture to try and complete that half an hour, but I was determined. I was going to do anything necessary to get better. In case you haven't noticed, not two days are alike. That is why it is very important to enhance and to repeat the same step until you are really comfortable.*

My feelings: There was burning when I first took it in. My hand and arm go stiff when I take my finger in. It feel as if my finger would move if I moved my arm and it would hurt a lot. I feel more pain while taking it out.

Day 5

Finger	Depth	Entries	Contraction (0-10)	Duration	
Index	1 node	8	5	30 min.	*As I discipline myself, my contractions become less and my exercise duration becomes longer. It felt as if I was doing better... It was very important for me to see this progress... I'm slowly starting to believe that I can do this.*

My feelings: Depending on the way I enter, I mean a bit higher, a bit left or right, the pain I feel changes. What am I going to do when the penis moves inside me? I can't move my finger at all when it's inside me. The contraction does not come when I put my finger inside but when I move it.

TABLES OF EXERCISE DIARIES

Day 6

Finger	Depth	Entries	Contraction (0-10)	Duration	
Index, Middle	1 node	20	4	45 min.	If you've noticed, I am still questioning future steps. Yes I was doing the exercises but I just couldn't imagine how I could do the further steps. Such thoughts are disaffecting...get them out of your mind. Just do your current homework, the rest will come. By the way, did you notice that the contractions are weakening as the number of entries increase? The more you increase the duration, the more the vagina gets used to entries. (It will be a huge mistake for me to move on to the next stage with my current scores. I am not ready for the second step yet. Don't skip steps before you are ready.)

My feelings: I noticed that the thing that provides my finger to remain inside is the fact that I keep my arm stiff. When I loosen my arm, the finger comes out by itself, it doesn't go in. The finger is small, the penis is thicker, I just can't understand how it could go in... I tried half of the exercises in kneeling position. It felt like I could take it in easier that way... The path inside me is not smooth, it is as if there are bumps in there. The way I stick my finger inside is what determines whether I feel pain or not. Sometimes it is somewhere, sometimes it doesn't. When I open my legs wide while taking my finger inside, the contraction loosens up and goes away.

Day 7

Finger	Depth	Entries	Contraction (0-10)	Duration	
Index	6 x one node, 2 x half	8	6	30 min.	While doing the exercises, if it happens to be a day when I feel bad, it would reflect on the exercises. It felt as if I was trying to dig a big hole with a pin. The first week is very important for the exercises, so keep your inner strength high. Your husband's support is very important here. It is his husbandly duty to be by your side, make him feel that. A loving man would not refrain from helping anyway. You may feel like you are going back at times, don't be disheartened ad keep going. You will be more comfortable at future stages.

My feelings: I take one node when I take my finger in for the first time. It tightens up and slowly pushes it out. It doesn't accept it.

Day 8

Finger	Depth	Entries	Contraction (0-10)	Duration	
Index	3 full nodes, 5 times half	8	8	55 min.	Again, a bad day and bad results. The first week is really hard... There nothing more difficult than fighting with yourself. You always try to evade, try to come up with excuses not to do the exercises. Don't even finish this week with a defeat... It becomes difficult to continue when your periods get in the way. So when you restart, start from one step back... You need to be comfortable first.

My feelings: I feel awful today. I don't want to do finger exercises.

Day 9

Finger	Depth	Entries	Contraction (0-10)	Duration	
Middle finger	1 node	6	7	45 min.	Here, the brain is fighting its last battle to resist. If I had given up at this stage, I would still have vaginismus today.

My feelings: My contractions have increased lately.

Day 10

Finger	Depth	Entries	Contraction (0-10)	Duration	
Middle, Index	1 node	8	5	45 min.	Here, the brain is fighting its last battle to resist. If I had given up at this stage, I would still have vaginismus today. My scores are still not enough to pass on to the second stage. But I can clearly say that I was almost flying during the next weeks. The first steps are really very difficult.

My feelings: My contractions have really increased lately. I went to the doctor and he told me my scores were not enough to pass to the second stage...

Day 11

Finger	Depth	Entries	Contraction (0-10)	Duration
Middle finger	1 node	16	3	35 min.

My feelings: I guess I'm doing better. The more I focus, the better it gets. I don't feel any pain today, just burning. I'm going to do this.

I just checked my diary and this is not my handwriting. My husband took notes for me... I dictated and he wrote them down, my love... What would I have done without you. I can't tell you how precious it was when you held my hand every time I said it was impossible... There are things I want to tell the men at this point; please support your wife. This is not an individual problem but a problem of couples.

Day 12

Finger	Depth	Entries	Contraction (0-10)	Duration
Middle finger	1 node	17	3	33 min.

My feelings: Yes, I think I feel more comfortable than yesterday but I still have the burning sensation. I should better increase this half an hour to one hour. I'm happy, I guess I'm showing progress.

As I wrote earlier, the principle of enhancement is very important for the exercises. We are not in a hurry. It is very important that we are patient, disciplined and orderly. The greatest mistake to do at these steps is to enter a delusion that you are fine and that you can move on to the next step. Don't move on to the next step before you feel the same comfort three days in a row. Some people dare to try future stages while still at the first steps. This will bring nothing but disappointment. Your efforts will be wasted...

Day 13

Finger	Depth	Entries	Contraction (0-10)	Duration
Middle finger	1 node	10	6	35 min.

My feelings: I'm doing bad again today. I'm demoralized. It doesn't happen when I force it.

Each day could be a different story during the exercises and it is very normal for you to feel that way during the initial stages. Therefore, you need to allocate sufficient time for the one finger, one node exercises. No hurries.

Day 14

Finger	Depth	Entries	Contraction (0-10)	Duration
Middle finger	1 node	22	5	80 min.

My feelings: Today I was so focused on increasing the number of entries and the duration that I ignored the contraction values and forced myself. Yes, I did it for longer but by ignoring the pain. I think I did wrong, I cab feel the chafe.

You should pay attention not to chafe while trying to prolong the exercises. One of the most important things here is not to do many entries but to them comfortably. Because if the number of entries increase and the contraction intensity increases at the same rate, it means that you are doing the exercises wrong. The rule is this; the number of entries should increase as you contractions decrease. The logic of forcing as much as possible to increase the number of entries is mistaken. We are trying to learn how not to feel pain, we aren't trying to enter the Guinness book of records!

Day 15

Finger	Depth	Entries	Contraction (0-10)	Duration
Index	1 node	17	6	25 min.

My feelings: I didn't do it for long today because I still have the chafing feeling. I won't force it again. It affects my motivation for the next day.

Forcing during exercises may backfire as much as hurrying. It is important to be determined and persevering at the one finger, one node stage but it is equally important not to pester yourself... Think of the exercises as games; if you condition them as homework, you could feel under pressure... By the way, a tip on exercises: if you push the vagina outside like you do while defecating, it makes entries easier.

TABLES OF EXERCISE DIARIES

IN THE FIRST WEEK, I WORKED FOR 266 MINUTES, DID 76 ENTRIES AND RECORDED A CONTRACTION SCORE OF 6.

IN THE SECOND WEEK, I WORKED FOR 295 MINUTES, DID 96 ENTRIES, RECORDED A CONTRACTION SCORE OF 5.

AS YOU CAN SEE, THESE RESULTS THAT I GOT IN FIFTEEN DAYS WERE NOT ENOUGH FOR MY DOCTOR TO ALLOW ME TO PASS TO THE NEXT STAGE.

TAKING THIS AS BASIS, YOU CAN ALSO HAVE AN IDEA ON WHETHER YOU ARE READY TO MOVE ON TO THE NEXT STAGE OR NOT.

HERE ARE THE VALUES THAT I RECORDED IN MY THIRD WEEK

WEEK 3

Day	Finger - Node(s)	Entries	Contraction (0-10)	Duration	
1	Index - 1 node	22	3	37 min.	If you pay attention, I was doing the exercises every day of the week. I think, if you've focused on this thing, the more you work, the more success you will have. I think it's worth distressing yourself for a period as short as three months.
2	I had guests, I couldn't do any				My values at the end of this week were sufficient to pass to the upper stage but I had done them for one more week because my appointment with the doctor was next week. Well, it worked out fine after all. I got better at it.
3	71 x Index - 2 nodes / 1 x Middle - 2 nodes	72	2	1 hour	Did you notice that I was only able to pass to the second node at the end of the second week?
4	11 x Index - 2 nodes / 24 x Index - Full length / 60 x Mid - Full length	95	0	1 hour	In the third week, I was very comfortable. So the two nodes and full length came automatically in the same week... and again, if you've noticed, as my contraction
5	60 x Index - Full length / 33 x Mid - Full length	93	0	1 hour	scores got lower, my entries skyrocketed! Frankly, my patience paid off ⑱
6	Index - Full length	64	2	40 min.	
7	Index - Full length	129	0	1 hour	

WEEK 4

Day	Finger - Node(s)	Entries	Contraction (0-10)	Duration	
1	Index - Full length	150	0	40 min.	The key to passing on to the next stage is getting your contraction score to two or less, rather than increasing your entry numbers. Of course, the number of entries shouldn't be that low. Anyway, when your contraction values decrease, the number of entries will
2	Index - Full length	100	0	35 min.	increase in parallel. Noticing this inverse correlation will give you an idea about moving to the upper stage.
3	76 x Index - Full length / 4 x Middle - Full length	80	1	35 min.	One of the mistakes done during the exercises (Especially during three-node entries) is to go on an exploration in there. Since we are not gynecologist candidates, we shouldn't go on an expedition to discover what is inside. We should not go on, "That's a cartilage,
4	Index - Full length	100	0	35 min.	here's a bone, oh what is this here..." and declare ourselves as abnormal creatures. Once you've learned how not to feel pain, pass on! No need for deep investigations. Our aim is
5	Index - Full length	120	0	35 min.	not to feel pain while something is going inside, not to reinvent the wheel.
6	I was sick, couldn't do any				As you can see, I was flying in week three. Yes, the first two weeks passed with distress and hardship but I didn't hurry to pass to stage two. Things came easily and quickly as I continued to exercise. When I called my doctor and told him, he had asked me to come
7	Index - Full length	150	0	30 min.	over for him to see my scores. And my scores were enough to move on to a new stage...

TABLES OF EXERCISE DIARIES

WEEK 5 — At this stage, while you do two-finger exercises in the first half hour, in the second half hour your husband makes one-finger trials first and then two-finger trials.

Scores for my solo two-finger exercises					Scores for our one-finger exercises with my husband					Comments
Day	Node(s) with two fingers	Entries	Contraction (0-10)	Duration (Mins)	Day	Node(s) with one fingers	Entries	Contraction (0-10)	Duration (Mins)	
1	1	30	6	30	1	1	50	4	30	This week, while the scores for exercises with my husband's finger were enough to move to the next stage, my solo scores were not. So we repeated the same exercises in the following week. You may experience an opposite situation. I mean, you can be comfortable with your own finger but not with your husband's finger. It may vary for each person.
2	1	35	6	30	2	1	70	3	30	
3	1	24	7	30	3	1	82	2	30	
4	1	35	5	30	4	2	90	0	40	
5	1	35	5	30	5	2	110	0	45	
6	1	40	4	30	6	2	115	0	45	
7	1	45	3	30	7	3	120	0	50	

WEEK 6 — (Eight days of menstruation period and the first examination by a gynecologist afterwards)

Day	Node	Entries	Contraction	Duration	Day	Node	Entries	Contraction	Duration	Comments
1	2	59	4	90	1	3	100	0	30	As you can see, this following week, things seem to be getting better... In the meanwhile, I had wanted to see a gynecologist now that I was feeling better. Frankly, I can't say that I was very comfortable but according to my doctor, there was a world of difference between my first visit and now. Actually, I didn't feel any pain but the fear was enough for me to have contractions. So, it's totally psychological... There is no pain if you are comfortable. When you menstruation period gets in between, you can start from one step back, with a warm-up round. As you may notice, I moved on to three-nodes because I was comfortable with my husband (see contraction values). One of the mistakes I did was being stubborn in increasing my number of entries. This is a mistake because it can cause chafes. Don't forget; no hurries. We are not trying to break a record.
2	2	52	4	55	2	3	100	1	30	
3	2	30	4	30	3	2 fingers, 1 node	30	3	30	
4	2	50	3	30	4	2 fingers, 1 node	110	1	30	
5	2	102	3	50	5	2 fingers, 1 node	110	0	20	
6	2	136	3	50	6	2 fingers, 1 node	160	1	30	
7	2	80	3	30	7	We couldn't try with my husband, he had work				

WEEK 7 — This week, we passed on to two fingers with my husband. For further enhancement, I continued my solo two-finger exercises as well and they were useful. My contractions are really less now.

Day	Node(s) with two fingers	Entries	Contraction (0-10)	Duration (Mins)	Day	Node(s) with two fingers	Entries	Contraction (0-10)	Duration (Mins)	Comments
1	2	80	3	45	1	1	145	1	30	As you may notice, in my solo two-finger exercises, even though there was no three-node step but I tried it anyway, out of curiosity. But I was mistaken because there is no need. This was good for nothing other than feeling my inside more and aversely effecting my concentration. The scores for my own finger exercises are enough for the next stage...
2	3	200	2	45	2	1	200	1	30	
3	3	200	2	30	3	2	60	3	30	
4	2	120	4	30	4	2	60	3	15	
5	2	87	2	40	5	2	77	4	30	
6	2	123	2	30	6	2	117	2	30	
7	2	175	0	30	7	2	165	3	30	

WEEK 8 — We continue our two-finger exercises with my husband.

Day	Node	Entries	Contraction	Duration	Comments
1	1	125	3	30	I am ready for penis trials now
2	2	115	2	30	
3	My husband was away, we couldn't try				
4	1	100	3	20	
5	2	240	0	30	
6	My husband was away, we couldn't try				
7	2	223	0	30	
8	2	185	0	30	
9	2	60	2	13	
My period again, one week pause					
1	2	120	0	20	
2	2	200	1	1	
3	2	130	2	2	
4	2	240	0	0	

Notes on the things I felt at the time: Two fingers were not as difficult as I had thought. Even I was surprised that I could take them simply with a contraction value of just two. In fact, I was so comfortable that I continued with two modes instead of one. I guess I'm slowly coming to the final ? I think the initial stages are more difficult. Once you get past them, the rest comes automatically.

In this stage of the exercise that you do with your husband, in the first half hour you place two of your fingers inside together while they are joined at the tips (Get the tips of your index and middle fingers together). It is enough to take in one node at first. Don't forget: Never force it. Wait until the contractions go away and you pull the fingers out as soon as they go away and put the fingers back in. After completing the first half hour by yourself, this time your husband tries entries with the same depth (Two fingers, one node).

I had gone to a gynecologist for the first time this week. By the way, there may be changes in your menstruation cycles because of the exercises, that is normal. It can happen due to the stress you are under. So when this happened, I built up all my courage and went to see a gynecologist for the first time. Even though I struggled during the vaginal examination, I had it anyway. The reason why I struggled was because of straining myself.

It is also normal for you to struggle in the exercises after the menstruation periods that get in the way. Give yourself time. Start from one step down and I am sure you'll get it together in no time.

VAGINISMUS DIARY 2

Hello Mr. Murat,

As per your request, I have written down everything that I went through since the beginning. I hope I can provide a bit of help for others. I am open to your suggestions. This is how I imagined my page...

My Vaginismus Diary

I had this problem for seven years. With the things it made me go through and the things it took from me, this illness had become the focal point of my life. Those who have the same problem will understand very well what I am trying to say. In such a situation, the most saddening thing is being left alone. You feel as lonely as you have never been... My first days passed by, thinking that I was going through something that no one else had ever experienced. This was an illness that nobody else suffered and it had found me. Everything was like a nightmare... At first, I couldn't believe that I was having this, and then I was alienated from life...I was twenty-two years old...all alone in this enormous city... At the time, my husband had a very busy work schedule, yet he was doing his best for me to get well.

We had heard the word vaginismus for the first time when we were one and a half years into our marriage. I had learned that I was not the only one in the World with this problem. Then we both tried to learn about this subject. Financial problems and being unable to find the right physician cost us many years. Years passed by, taking a lot away from me. I was in love with my husband but I had begun loathing sex. I didn't want to have any kind of sexuality with my husband, I was repulsed by it... I hated being a woman. Other than sex, we were very happy with my husband... We were madly in love with each other, and we still are...

Then we moved to a bigger city to receive treatment and to find a good physician, and we started seeing a psychiatrist. I began feeling better after each therapy... I was in a great battle with myself, trying to change my thoughts. I kept on reading, investigating, praying... I realized that I didn't know my organ at all, that I had ignored it for years, rejected it... I have fought with myself a lot since that time until now. You can't change just like that, you can't get better thoughts to replace the negative ones so easily.

But when you want…when you make an effort…gigantic mountains turn into tiny hills…

During the day, I was instilling myself with positive thoughts at certain times when I was alone. I was trying to build positive dreams, to get rid of the negativities… Days went by this way… It had been six months since the beginning of the therapy… I didn't hate sex any more… The only thing I had not been able to get over was the fear of the penis… I had come to a deadlock… I could not even pass to the trial stages; that was how afraid I was… Just as I was giving up hope, I found the website and the group… And when I got to know Mr. Murat, I made up my mind. I was going to see him. I stopped going to the psychiatrist. I was feeling much better in the group, I was feeling happy with the supports of my friends there who had been successful. I was not going to give up… And most importantly, I was not feeling lonely… I began doing finger exercises and managed them in a period as short as eight days. With each finger exercise you realize this; "My vagina is not a closed area as I thought it was! I understand that the vagina is a highly elastic organ and I have control over it!"

When I was really comfortable with the finger, we moved to the penis stage… One night, I took the penis inside under my control… Everything happened so suddenly… There was no pain! The happiness I felt at that time is indescribable! I looked into my husband's eyes… We never gave up on loving each other… We continued to share life with everything it brought us… On the next night, I had contractions at the first try… It was as if all the old thoughts had rushed back into my head. I suddenly withdrew myself. I felt as if I had been caught in a meaningless whirlpool of fear.

"I HAD BEEN SUCCESSFUL BUT MY BRAIN STILL DID NOT BELIEVE THE THING THAT MY BODY BELIEVED!"

It was either give up or go on… With the support I received from Mr. Murat and from the group, I went on… Everything went better in our next trial and the others that followed… I understood that there is nothing the brain can't do!

I had read it somewhere, "Owning the thing you have just learned depends on you experiencing it right then." There may be obstacles in front of you but a person should be able to create solutions rather than solutionlessness. Every person's time frame in defeating vaginismus may be different; everyone has different reactions. I believe that everyone should create her own program, without falling apart from the existing exercise program.

By listening to the voice inside yourself and by trying to apply what you already have to the program, you should draw your own path to success… Don't wait for miracles! You are the miracle…

Change your negative thoughts…
Don't delay…
Don't give up…
Take action…
Be decisive…
And dream…

This is my story. My next goal is to help you all. I know what you are going through and more importantly, I can understand you… Don't be afraid and don't refrain from seeking help… We are not alone any more…

Exercises

My advice to those who will do the exercises is to prepare themselves for it. You need to let yourself into the program calmly in a comfortable environment. Once you realize that you are doing something for yourself, this could turn into a fun activity for you. Don't forget that you are doing this because you want to… There may be times when you have difficulty; that is very normal… Nobody is expecting you to run before you learn to crawl, anyway… Be calm

1. First step, getting to know the vagina with a mirror and touching it. You can do this as much as you like and increase your knowledge by touching. At this point, I suggest you to read books that will help you learn about the anatomy of your vagina. As you learn more about your body, it will become easier for you to be cleared of the false notions in your head. Do research. You will see that you will get rid of myths as you learn.

2. The touching stage.
- Dressed touching (Except genital areas)
- Undressed touching (Except genital areas)
- Undressed touching (Including genital areas)
- Undressed touching (Genital areas in particular)

Firstly, you touch each other in turns with your husband while you are clothed, standing up and in a massaging manner. The aim of caressing each other's bodies and giving pleasure is to increase your sensitivities toward each other and to make each other take more pleasure with sensual contact. In later steps, you can do the same while sitting or lying down. You need to do each of the above for four to five minutes.

3. Massage stage.

You will do this to each other's front and back sides with baby oil. This is an application that is a massage done by drawing small circles with your hand, with slight pressure, and intensify it at the areas where you take most pleasure. Here, you will learn to completely relax your body. You will direct your spouse toward the areas you like best. Then your husband will place his hand on your vagina for fifteen minutes. While totally under your control, you will be getting used to a foreign object in that area. As sexual intercourse is not advised at this stage, the woman will comfortably let herself go with the flow.

You need to repeat these stages as much as possible, this way you will also be curing frigidity, if you have it.

4. Finger Exercises (I'll explain it shortly for those who may not know).

The goal in finger exercises is to understand that something can go in there and to train, accustom the muscles there by moving in and out… This way, we take control of our muscles and systemically change the reflex there. When the person sticks her finger in her vagina, she understands that the vagina is not a closed place as she had imagined! This thought helps her get over the other stages more easily. First we take in any finger that we feel comfortable with, up to the first node… Water-based gels may be used as lubricant.

One finger, one node: We work at this stage until we are totally comfortable. No passing on to the next step before becoming absolutely comfortable… It could take a few days, or a week, or ten days… You must understand yourself well… Wait if you have contractions, and when they go away, take your finger out and continue. If you don't have any contractions, there is no need to wait… You try over and over again.

One finger, two nodes: This is the same; wait if you have contractions, if not, take it out and repeat. You should move on to the next step only after you are completely comfortable…

One finger, three nodes: This step is the same, too… Wait if you have contractions, if not, take it out and repeat… You already got the hang of it; we do it until we are fully comfortable. There is no need to pester ourself; the important thing is to train our muscles. Don't start two finger exercises before you are absolutely comfortable.

Two fingers, one node: We try to take in our index and middle fingers at the same time, but only up to one node. This step could feel more difficult than the others, but don't panic! You don't need to hurry, since the aim is just to train the muscles there. You couldn't do it in your first try? Try again without giving up… We need to put both fingers in at the same time. The same rule applies to this step too; don't move on to the next step before feeling absolutely comfortable. We wait when we have contractions, we continue when they pass… We do it over and over again… Until we are really really comfortable.

Two fingers, two nodes: This will be the same. The rule is simple; wait when contracting, take out when it's gone and repeat.

Two fingers, three nodes: This is also the same… You will do this step with the same logic… Now you have trained the muscles there and you are very close to the result.

Now it is time for your husband's finger… You will repeat the steps above with him one by one… If you do this after being very comfortable with your own finger, this will not be too difficult…

But still, some women may have difficulty with her husband's finger… Such people can move on to the penis stage after getting really comfortable with their own two fingers. Think of the penis as a finger and take in the tip first. Then you will take half, and then the whole… Step by step, I mean…

Finger exercises are not as difficult as you may think. You will see for yourself after you start doing them. Once you have started, the rest will come on its own…

The important thing is to be determined…

Kegel Exercises

At the pelvis area, I mean under the pubis bone, there are muscles around the vagina entrance, and these are called pelvic muscles. These are the muscles moved by the woman while urinating… These muscles are also those that help with retention, intercourse, orgasm and childbirth…

Pay attention to what muscles you are using when you stop your urination halfway. Or place a finger inside your vagina and squeeze… These are the muscles that we will work on.

1. During the exercise, clamp your pelvic floor muscles for ten seconds. And give a ten-second break… Do this consecutively for five or ten times. Continue to breathe normally during the exercise and just make sure that your pelvic muscles are working…
2. Lie down on your back and slightly separate your knees. Concentrate on your vaginal muscles and slowly pull your pelvic muscles upward. This way, the vagina entrance becomes slightly turned upward, ready for intercourse. You may find it difficult at first but you will understand how you need to do it as you try… In the meanwhile, make sure that you don't

clamp your stomach or your hip muscles. Count to ten and relax. Repeat for a few times. I suggest you to do this every day. These are exercises that will especially benefit those who have intense contractions. This way, you learn how to control your muscles[11].

With love,
Nickname, Deniz.

As you can see, in classical treatments, everything is practiced by doing a lot of repetitions and by dividing into the smallest pieces. The transition to the penis is also done in pieces.

As you will see in the following pages, with The Dr. Ulusoy Method in vaginismus treatment, the result is obtained in three phases and in one and a half days on average. The transition to the penis is done directly. The utilization of appropriate hypnosis techniques is what lies beneath obtaining results in such short time.

---

(11) **Author's note**: Deniz' diary also comprises of classical treatment. It contains Kegel Exercises. As said earlier, the vagina is loose in the vaginismus seen in Turkish women. So, there is no need for Kegel Exercises.

SEX POSITIONS

It is possible to describe many sex positions. They could be classified as simple, intermediate and advanced. Couples could start from the simple positions and move on to advanced positions. Due to the contents of our book, we have only touched upon the positions that are simple and that ease the first penis – vagina coupling. There are books for couples who wish to try advanced positions at future stages to embark on a journey in discovering different pleasures. After succeeding in the treatment, my advice to couples is to learn together from books about different positions that are shaped with love games and try them, rather than going on with a monotonous sex life and limited number of positions.

PICTURES OF THE PENIS
EXPERIENCE AND SEX POSITIONS

FİRST PENİS ENTRANCE

Below, you can see a position with the woman on top, placing the penis into the vagina entrance and taking the penis inside gradually by sitting on it. The woman has total control.

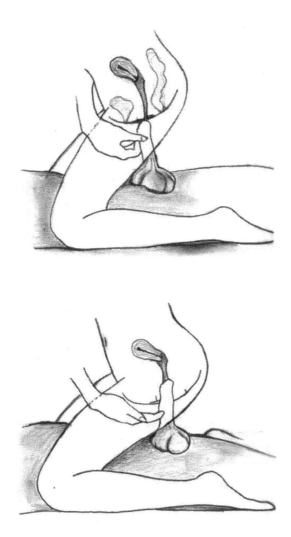

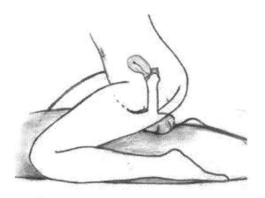

Pic-7-8-9: Taken from the book Completely Overcome Vaginismus, modified and redrawn by A. Ayşe Yalçındağ

Below is a raised surface. It is a balanced position for both the man and the woman as the penis and vagina are at the same level and the woman's legs are around the man's waist. It allows the man to steer by seeing. The man has control.

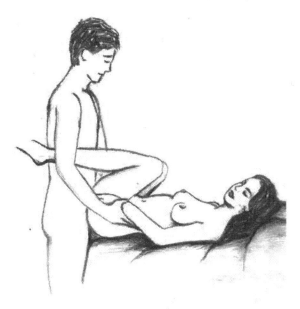

Pic-10: Taken from the book *Sexual Reflexology-Dharma Publications*, modified and redrawn by A. Ayşe Altındağ

Below is a position in which the woman is down on her knees and elbows, and where the man places the penis into the vagina from behind. This position is especially suitable for patients who cannot feel comfortable with transferring the authority to the man. Since intercourse during an approach from the behind takes place out of the woman's line of sight, she feels relatively more comfortable. The man is in control.

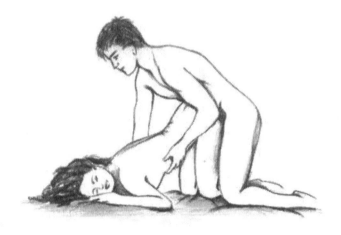

Pic-11: Taken from the book *Sexual Reflexology-Dharma Publications,* modified and redrawn by A. Ayşe Altındağ

In the position below, the man is in lying position and the woman is sitting on her knees, as if riding a horse, and she takes the penis inside while face-to-face with the man. The woman has total control.

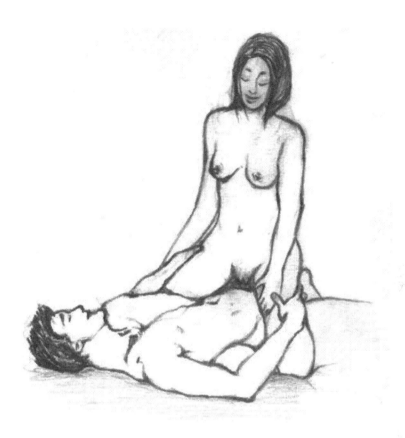

Pic-12: Taken from the book *Sexual Reflexology-Dharma Publications*, modified and redrawn by A. Ayşe Altındağ

Below is the position where the man is in lying position and the woman is squatting with her back toward the man. The man is supporting the woman from her hips and the couple is inserting the penis inside in harmony. The woman and man have joint control.

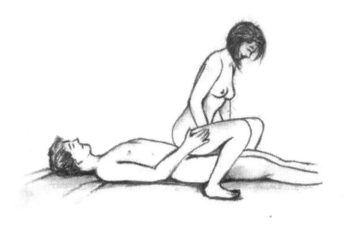

Pic-13: Taken from the book *Sexual Reflexology-Dharma Publications,*
modified and redrawn by A. Ayşe Altındağ

Below, the woman wraps her legs around the man's waist while she lies on her back and the man is on his knees. The man is in control.

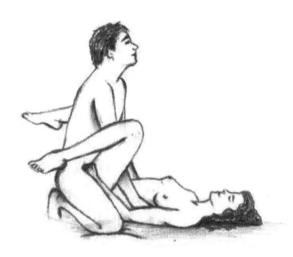

Pic-14: Taken from the book *Sexual Reflexology-Dharma Publications,*
modified and redrawn by A. Ayşe Altındağ

Below, the woman is on her back with her knees drawn to her belly and the man is on his knees. The man is in control.

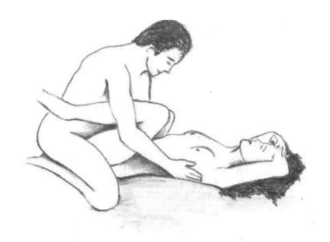

Pic-15: Taken from the book *Sexual Reflexology-Dharma Publications,*
modified and redrawn by A. Ayşe Altındağ

In the below position, the woman is lying on her back with her legs bent
from her knees and her soles touching the ground while the man is on his
knees. The man is in control. The woman is more balanced because her soles
are touching the ground.

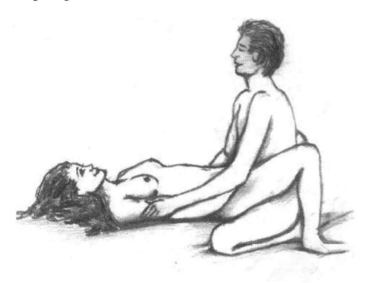

Pic-16: Taken from the book *Sexual Reflexology-Dharma Publications,*
modified and redrawn by A. Ayşe Altındağ

Below, the man is lying down and the woman is squatting with her face
toward the man. The woman has control.

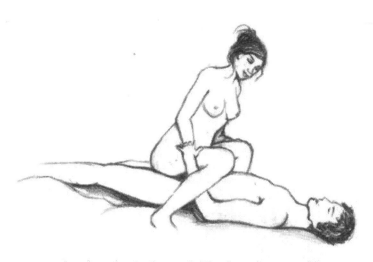

Pic-17: Taken from the book *Sexual Reflexology-Dharma Publications,* modified and redrawn by A. Ayşe Altındağ

Below is a position where the man is half-seated and where the woman is on her knees with her back turned to the man as she holds his ankles. The man is in control.

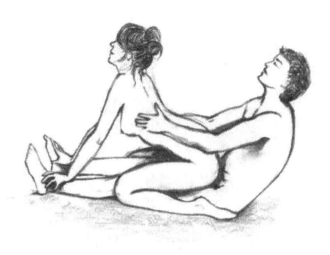

Pic-18: Taken from the book *Sexual Reflexology-Dharma Publications,* modified and redrawn by A. Ayşe Altındağ

SAMPLE CASES FROM THE 146 WOMEN WHO SOLVED THEIR VAGINISMUS PROBLEM WITH THE FREE SUPPORT I PROVIDED FOR TWELVE MONTHS OVER YAHOO! GROUPS DURING THE YEARS 2005 AND 2006

I would like to share some of the e-mails from the cases solved in our Yahoo group. All the names and cities in the following e-mails have been taken out in a way that the cases cannot be identified. These vaginismus patients, who had not received any treatment at all or who had been to classical treatments, are telling their success stories within the dynamics of the group. At the same time, these will reveal the things that are happening in classical treatment.

Sample Case 1

Hello Everybody,

I want to tell you that I succeeded, too. After the finger exercises that lasted about two months, I passed the penis stage, too. I had no difficulties at the final stages of finger exercises. I was easily taking two fingers inside, with gel of course… Perseverance is very important my friends… And self-confidence… As I go to work during the day, I could only do the finger exercises at night before going to bed. On a similar night, I asked my husband for it. Would I be able to take his finger? I mean, something other than myself, other than my own finger…

I took in my husband's finger. Without any problems. One can guide herself while taking in her own finger but this is relatively less with your husband's finger… The control somewhat passes to the husband's finger… "Why not?" I thought and passed on to the penis stage, gathering my courage… Now my husband doesn't go inside by himself. I mean, intercourse doesn't come after a lustful foreplay. I take the penis inside. Then he goes on… I guess I'll get past that in time.

I have a little anxiety when he first goes inside me. There is almost no pain. It just feels like I need to use the bathroom. But that passes later. As my husband slowly goes in and out, I feel that I'm taking pleasure.

I must tell my friends, who have gone past the finger stages, that they should not fear the penis stage. Believe me; it is not what we make of it. Take control with the penis, too. Just as I did… You place it inside yourself. But not in a trice… The rest will come on its own. While I was urinating after the first intercourse, I felt some burning inside. But that is gone now. I'm thinking about the other things I felt… There is a slight burning at first entry but don't ever stop. Tell yourself to keep on… Go on, don't give up… We have so many other pains; we cut our finger or have an injection. Believe me; this is not as painful… We are having problems because we have psychologically conditioned ourselves. And it is a reality that your husband's support, his motivation during intercourse, the words he says are very important… I don't know but these things gave me strength. Being his woman… Right now, the only thing I want is to live that moment after sex. I mean, letting go to the flow… To feel my husband completely inside me, rather than in my hand… I wish everyone gets it easy. I hope we all reach the happiness we strive for… Like I said; don't give up, believe in yourself and always persevere.

With love…

Sample Case 2

I DID IT!

Hello everybody. I haven't been able to write anything for a long time. I just made do by following the things you had written, your advices and your experiences. I was in a difficult, painful period. My head was so confused. As I had said, I am married for two years and I was suffocated by living with this problem. I was ashamed, I couldn't tell anyone, I felt like a sad sack with my husband, I was eating myself up, thinking why I was unable to something that everyone else was doing, and many other things… You already know and go through the same things. But one month ago, I really decided to take care of this problem and went to a psychologist. Everything was very difficult at first. I was having a lot of trouble with sharing my problem. My psychologist constantly gave me inspiration on getting to know my vagina. He asked me to do online research about this. And I did so. I learned a lot of things about my vagina that I hadn't known before. Then I clarified the things I had learned first with my hand and then by making examinations on the outer surface of my vagina in front of a mirror. This way, I was somewhat able to break the ice between my vagina and myself. Then I coincidentally found this web site. This really relieved me a lot because so many people were having the same problem and our struggles were the same. I was not alone! This enabled me to share my problems with my psychologist more easily. I thank you all and especially Mr. Murat for this.

In the meanwhile, I continued my research. I examined the vagina's ability to expand, the structures of the hymen. I was relieved and all, but how was the entrance going to be? I was very scared, thinking, "What if I fail again?" The posts were always talking about the necessity of finger exercises but it devastated me to even think about it. I could never do it. I was not ready for that at all. The finger felt so repulsive to me. Then I sat down and thought, and then I decided that I preferred the penis to the finger. My husband and I hadn't made love for three weeks as per my psychologist's advice. Now that my self-confidence was building up, I decided to try. We tried and I could take the penis halfway inside... It was the first time we had made so much progress and we were very happy. But the same thing happened in the next two-three trials. It felt as if there was a wall and it could not go any further. This broke my confidence a lot. I was demoralized. Then, thanks to therapy, I was able to pull myself together. I tried to educate myself on how I could get rid of the confusion in my head during sex. This was very easy and I was going to do it. That was what I kept on thinking.

And today, everything happened by itself! I took my husband's penis and placed it inside my vagina. I moved it further and it slid inside like soap. The pain was not as bad as I had thought. Everything was so smooth. I remember crying with happiness at the time.

You will manage it, too. Please believe that. Just believe and don't fear. First of all, don't be a stranger to your vagina, get to know it. Then rule over your brain. If the method suitable for you is finger exercises, do them. But most importantly, change your thoughts. I DID IT SO BELIEVE ME; YOU CAN DO IT TOO...

I managed it but the problems are not gone yet. The penis goes inside very easily but I feel unbearable pains when the in and out motion begins. I start to have contractions again. I wonder if this is normal at the beginning. The only thing I have managed is being on top and going back and forth slowly. I can't manage any other position than this one. I guess I'm starting to get demoralized again!

Sample Case 3

Hello Everyone,

We are almost in a dream right now. We have been married for two and a half years. Apparently we have spent one and a half years in vain, thinking that we could overcome the vaginismus problem on our own. We had decided to receive treatment and we had started seeing a physician. My wife was very hopeless. Earlier, she could not dare look at it, let alone touch it. It took her one month just to get started with the finger exercises. But then everything progressed gradually. We did everything the doctor told us. During our treatment, we met this group. We felt we were not alone when we saw all these people sharing the same things. We succeeded three and a half months ago. And during one month of this period, we were able to have intercourse with help of baby oil. Then we thought that it could harm the baby so we stopped suing any substances. Apparently, this way it is more beautiful, more slippery and more special. Now my wife is one-month pregnant. WE ARE EXPECTING A BABY. We wanted to share this wonderful news with you because this group was very helpful for us during treatment. We took strength from your messages.

We hope that all of you can overcome this problem in a short time. Truly, everything is in the person's head. We will pray for you. May God bestow this on everyone.

Sample Case 3

Hello Doctor,

First of all, we would like to thank you and our friends in the group. We did our fifteen-day homework and I supported my wife a great deal. She was extremely influenced by the posts that you and the others shared in the group and she was determined to do it. We did our homework with great perseverance. In the end, she felt regret for having waited in vain for five years. May God bless you, Doctor. I hope God always keeps sensitive and understanding people like you there for people who do not have the financial means. We thank you once again for your support, and we wish you success in your studies. We will never ever forget you. WE MADE IT... WE MADE IT... WE MADE IT...

Best regards, doctor.

Sample Case 4

Hello people, although I didn't write much, I kept following the mails. And I took help from a psychologist for a while. The finger exercises had been finished months ago and we had been scared even to try intercourse.

Last night, it happened on its own. Moreover, may husband ejaculated inside me. I didn't get much pleasure because of the contractions but it is a nice feeling. By the way, I am married for six years. "Was this all that I waited for all these years?" I said to myself... Believe me; it is very easy.

Mr. Murat, it was just that I had a lot of bleeding. It was over in a few hours but I bled a lot, perhaps it was because of the contractions. What could be the reason? I didn't feel a lot of pain. I'm curious; can I do it again?

Try; don't give up halfway. It is very easy. I thank everyone very much...

Sample Case 5

Hello Doctor and Friends,

I had just joined the group while I was at the one finger, one node stage and under physician supervision. Later on, I kept following the group. The homeworks that my doctor gave me were in accordance with the diaries and posts in the group. I never could have thought that I could succeed. I was very jealous of the "I did it" e-mails. But on Saturday, about two months after starting treatment, *I did it too*.

I, who has a very low pain threshold and who has even avoided injections, didn't feel any pain at all. I thank everyone who has sent posts in this group, and I also thank you Doctor for creating such a group. Until one week ago, I was able to take in my husband's two fingers and three nodes very easily. And when we finally went to the doctor on Thursday, he said we could try the penis stage now. I was scared for a while and I didn't try it for two days. But in our first trial, I saw that it was easier than the fingers and now I don't even need to go to a doctor because I can do it easily, even without gel. I suggest everyone to do her homework regularly. AND IN THE END, I MANAGED. It was for nothing that I had struggled for four years.

Sample Case 6

I did it too, hooray!

This is totally a psychological problem. It is truly about being ready for intercourse and wanting it. We create the pain in our brains. Before getting married, I was asking almost everyone around me about the pain. I groomed this question in my mind for years and turned it into a problem. I followed the mails for two months. "I can do it, I can do it too," I kept on saying to myself and I did! We tried four more times after the first one and I was successful in three of them. ☺ I still haven't overcome my problem about taking pleasure but with the help of God, I'm going to get over that too.

During the intercourse, I am still unable to believe that I managed it so I can't concentrate and take pleasure…

In the e-mails, people used to write that if they did it, everyone could do it. Now I am saying the same thing; if I did it, all of you can…

Believe me; it is just a teeny-weeny sting, that's all… It's not worth waiting for that… It is not worth upsetting yourself… I wish everyone success from the bottom of my heart… God is on our side, don't forget that and let's all pray for each other… Believing is halfway to success; believe that you can do it first…

CHAPTER 5

USEFUL INFORMATION

This chapter contains additional readings.

INTERVIEW WITH
DR. MURAT ULUSOY ON
VAGINISMUS

Q: How do you treat vaginismus?

A: I consider three main factors while treating vaginismus.
1. Education
2. Investigating for problems with the vagina (We check to see whether something can enter or not, due contractions at the lower vagina muscles. If something can go in, can the vagina adapt to the diameter and thickness?)
3. Working on mind-body relaxation with clinical hypnosis in order to replace the contractions that occur during intercourse (Pushing spouse away involuntarily, withdrawal, contracting and closing legs) with relaxation via therapy. I provide a therapy approach that targets the causes of the patient's vaginismus.

Q: What is the difference from the classical methods?

A: Classical vaginismus treatments have an approach that lasts twelve weeks with weekly meetings. It is carried out with education, sexual prohibitions, homework on getting to know the body and also on the vagina. The fact that the treatment duration is long may cause the patient to drift away from treatment, or she could complete her homework but still be unable to have intercourse. Because although intercourse is anticipated after the education and homeworks are completed, there is also a group of patients that are referred to as *those who are able to take things inside but who cannot take the penis due to physical contractions*, as mentioned in my classification of vaginismus types.

At this point, it could be a good idea to take a look at our vaginismus classification for better understanding of the matter.

Classification of Vaginismus Patients (Dr. Ulusoy, 2018)

1. Those who cannot touch the labia majora or labia minora, or in between (Outer genitalia).
2. Those who can touch the outer genital area but not inside the vagina.
3. Those who can touch the outer genitalia and the vagina and can direct fingers inside, but who cannot have the penis experience.
4. Those who are in one of the three groups mentioned above and who do not have contractions, but who cannot allow the penis inside (Those with hip problems, breathing control problems or with problems of transferring of authority).
5. Those who are in one of the first three groups mentioned above and who have internal or external contractions ranging from minor to severe, and who cannot take in the penis.

As seen, various categories appear when we talk about vaginismus. The factors listed below also have effect on the woman at different proportions, so the vaginismus illness almost resembles an ivy.

1. The woman's own character patterns (i.e. panic attack, obsession, perfectionist structure, phobic and afraid of everything…).
2. Lack of sexual education and knowledge.
3. Physical differences between man and woman.
4. Cognitive, behavioral, dynamic and existentialistic factors.

Therefore, the vaginismus treatment should be planned by taking into consideration all these details.

At the same time, the *woman-man-therapist* trivet should be on solid ground. If one of the legs of the trivet is problematic, disruptions in the treatment will be inevitable.

The most important differences between our treatment and classical treatments are the following.

1. The treatment duration is less (One and a half days on average)
2. The success of clinical hypnosis in replacing physical contractions with relaxation

3. The fact that the therapy is directed toward quick learning with clinical hypnosis (Clinical hypnosis acts as a catalyst in the treatment)
4. The ability of clinical hypnosis to make homework more doable (The weakest point of classical treatments is the homework not being done)
5. During the treatment period, it is impossible to deny the effectiveness of clinical hypnosis sessions in vaginismus therapy according to the formulation that is based on cognitive, behaviorist, dynamic and existentialist structures that are among the vaginismus ethiology.
6. The fact that, with hypnosis and Holotropic Breathwork, we provide feedback-assisted control and relaxation at the Psoas Muscles that are the main factor in the ethiology.

Q: Is hypnosis the only method that you apply? Why do you use hypnosis?

A: In vaginismus treatment, I use clinical hypnosis together with cognitive and behaviorist treatments. The cognitive method and clinical hypnosis make it possible for us to resolve the perceptive distortions that create the problem at the mind, and also to create correct perceptions about intercourse in the mind. And with the behaviorist treatment, we do a short-term study to find out if something can enter the vagina, if the diameter can be tolerated, or if there is any problem with the hymen -physical problems- and we treat the problems, if any.

Q: What is the benefit of hypnosis?

A: Clinical hypnosis does the same job as an enzyme/catalyst does in a reaction.
1. It removes the mental resistances and eases learning
2. It makes it possible to do the homework that could not be done
3. It enables us to replace the contractions with relaxation
4. It speeds up and eases vaginismus treatment

Q: Why is it not enough to talk to the patients and give them homework in classical treatments?

A: There are resistances in our minds. While it is easy to talk to some patients (Vaginismus cases based on cognitive reasons, perceptive distortions and structures) and make them do their homework, it is not possible to reach other patients (Vaginismus cases based on behaviorist, dynamic and existentialist reasons) this way. The information that reaches the conscious is reflected by the resistance like a mirror, and the information is not able to penetrate into the subconscious to create change. Here, this is the point where clinical hypnosis comes in.

Q: Do you apply hypnosis only to women? What is the man's part in this treatment?

A: Our main concentration in vaginismus treatment is the woman, the owner of the problem. But in a good treatment, the triple harmony between the man, the woman and the therapist is required. Just like a triplet, all three need to be on solid ground.

The things that the man need to are the following.

1. Not to leave the problem to be solved in time
2. To support the woman for treatment
3. Not to blame his spouse for the vaginismus problem
4. To always be there for his spouse during treatment, to join in the education and treatment.

And in cases which I define as *The Seesaw Effect,* when the man faces an erection problem after the woman become able to have intercourse after therapy, we are able to support him within medical processes.

Q: Are there countries in the World that commonly use this method?

A: Around the World, there are places and therapist that apply cognitive or cognitive + behaviorist treatments, or solely hypnotherapy, or treatments that are a combination of all. But it must be pointed out that vaginismus ethiology (Reasons) vary according to cultures and personality structures. Therefore, the therapist needs to know the literature and be aware of the culture-specific differences and personality structures.

Q: In which congresses have you made presentations on the subject? What were these presentations about?

A: So far, I have made presentations at the national and international medical hypnosis congresses, 2011 European Hypnosis Congress, First and Second International Anatolia Sexual Health and Neuroscience Congress, International Asia Hypnosis Congress. A brief list is as follows.

•   2004 - Poster presentation on The Effectiveness of Hypnotherapy in Vaginismus Treatment during the 1st Medical Hypnosis Congress at Istanbul Yeditepe University with national and international attendance.

- 2005 - During the 2nd Medical Hypnosis Congress at Istanbul Yeditepe University with local and foreign attendance, I made the declaration that the "Seesaw Effect" is the secondary erection problem that can be seen in the man during vaginismus treatment, and that visualization should be used as the final step of the treatment and that this has been given the name "Simulation Method."
- 2006 - At the 3rd Medical Hypnosis Congress I declared that the average number of sessions has been reduced to 3.6 by using the *Maya Technique*.
- 2008 - I participated in the 5th Medical Hypnosis Congress with verbal presentation "Dr. Ulusoy Method in Vaginismus Treatment" at Istanbul Aydın University.
- 2009 - I provided presentation on "Main Factors Influencing Vaginismus Treatment; twenty main causes and four new definitions" at the 6th International Medical Hypnosis Congress at Istanbul Aydın University.
- 2011 - I provided presentation on "Dr. Ulusoy Hypnosis Induction Technique" and "Dr. Ulusoy Vaginismus Treatment Method" and shared retrospective analysis and survey results for 450 cases at the 12th ESH (European Hypnosis Congress) Congress at Istanbul Aydın University; thus reducing the treatment duration to twenty-four hours.
- 2012 - I provided verbal presentation on "Weight and Hypnosis," "Vaginismus Treatment" and "Dr. Ulusoy Hypnosis Induction Technique" at the 8th International Medical Hypnosis Congress at Üsküdar University.
- 2015 - I provided a verbal presentation and workshop for "Three phases and one and a half days in Vaginismus Treatment – Dr. Ulusoy Method" and the "5 – BK Model" at the International Anatolian Twin Congress On Neuroscience and Sexual Health in Istanbul in 2015.
- 2018 - I provided presentation on "Hypnosis in Vaginismus and Psoas Muscles" at 11th Congress of Turkish Hypnosis Association.
- 2019 - I provided verbal presentation on "Hypnosis for Vaginismus and the Psoas Muscle" at the 1st Asia Hypnosis Congress in Iran and another presentation on "Hypnosis for Vaginismus and the Psoas Muscle" at the 2nd Anatolia Sexual Health and Neuroscience Congress.

Q: Your patients have created an online fan club and they speak highly of you. What is the secret of your success?

A: I could summarize the secret of success in a few items.

1. Working according to cultural differences and personality characteristics.
2. Actively using clinical hypnosis.
3. Being in complete communication with the patient before (After appointment), during and after the treatment, and doing follow-up.
4. Making each patient feel special and providing her with special care during the average one and a half days of treatment -independent of sessions- in a problem-focused and solution-oriented way, and not taking other patients in between.
5. Therapeutic collaboration with the patient is difficult. It is not easy. The therapist's personality is important at this point; his character, humanitarianism, his potential to accept his patient as she is, his capability to love, his desire to help the person sitting across from him, his ability to approach without judging or condemning, his feelings of compassion and affection...
6. Using a good combination of treatment methods and approaches, helping my patient to focus on the treatment while easing her vaginismus treatment.

Q: Where do the patients come from? How do they find out about you?

A: We receive patients from many cities around Turkey. If you compare them with the population, Istanbul, Ankara, Izmir, Bursa, Konya and Antalya lead the way. And from abroad, we receive patients from the US, Europe, Middle East, Far East, Russia and African countries. They hear about mostly while doing online research. And in recent years, patients come with the direct advisements of our healed patients on online forums. I also witness that patients also advise us to their relatives, friends or even with people they have just met after finding out about their problem. Other than these, my colleagues also refer patients to us.

Q: What is your area of expertise?

A: I am a graduate of Thrace University Faculty of Medicine. I have been working on hypnosis and hypnotherapy since 1991. And since the early 2000s, I am involved with hypnosis trainings and congresses. I also completed a two-year psychotherapy education. I have a master's degree in clinical psychology.

I have received trainings on family counseling and sexual therapy. I chose vaginismus as my field of study and I have been working solely in this field since 2004. Medical science is an art. You try to perform your job in the best way possible. This is what every physician tries to do. The important thing is obtaining a high success rate in treatment as well as providing the patient's happiness and satisfaction.

Q: In how many days do you complete the treatment? Is a weekend enough? Why did you choose the town of Kuşadası?

A: The average time for success in our treatment is one and a half days (2011 ESH Congress presentation). We meet with our patient three times during the day, and after seeing her one last time the following morning, we come to the point where we can direct her toward intercourse. As most of our patients are from out of town, we ask them to add another day and a half just to have provision for their personality structures and for the risks in the treatment, so they are asked to spend three days at Kuşadası. In terms of weekends, if we take the patient on Friday morning, her problem will be solved by Saturday noon. If we have problems during treatment, this could last until Sunday.

I had worked in Nazilli Province before. Later, I chose a touristic town due to requests from my patients. Our patients come with the concept of *Treatment – Vacation – Honeymoon*. Besides, Kuşadası is a town that is easily reached by road or by air.

Q: Apparently you meet your patients and check them into the hotel… Could you elaborate some more?

A: Yes. The essence of the matter is being able to provide attention and patient satisfaction in the best way possible. You are coming to a foreign place, you have reservations and distress about your illness. In this case, we need to be with you as much as possible and support you. This is why our courtesy van picks our patient up and we help them check into the hotel. Our guest is given a special room with sea view by our contracted hotel -all the hotels we suggest are by seafront. Our treatment center is right next door to the hotel and I personally meet the patient during the day and we start the treatment process.

And at the end of our interview, we would like to share a letter from one of Dr. Ulusoy's patients which summarizes vaginismus and its treatment

I DID IIIIIITTTTTT!

I had promised myself that I would right a big *I did it.* Of course I will put the same writing on the online forum so that my friends there will not have a hard time trying fingers or candles, etc. so that they don't worry themselves…

I still can't believe how it happened but it happened, and I was able to do everything on my own. In our Doctor's words; I was not unconscious, nobody drugged me, I did it on my own. ☺

Dear vaginismus women, this letter is for you. Please read it.

For three years, I had been crying myself to sleep almost every night and I would thank God for the arrival of morning. And the next evening, the same things would repeat. Think about it, I tried to pass the days hoping that someone would come to visit, or that we would go somewhere, or that my husband would come home late, etc. But how much more could I delay it?

When tension starts, it doesn't end so easily. We were running out of patience for each other and we had begun getting annoyed with each other with the smallest of problems…

I tried a lot of things for the solution. I went to all them with belief but I could not get any results because in some cases, the doctors' approaches were wrong (Such as; this is very simple… Everything is normal; there is no obstacle for you not to do it… We have a package program; it will be over in three months or in one-two years… You can do it if we remove your hymen and you will need psychological treatment if you can't do it, etc.)

I had been following our good doctor for a long time. I had been reading all the messages since October and when finally our marriage began to fall apart, I made my decision and made an appointment.

I was able to do the thing, which had felt absolutely impossible on the first day. And in the end, I DID IT…

I still can't believe I am writing this.

The questions in my life before going to Dr. Ulusoy were,
- Why me?
- All women can do it, what am I lacking?
- Did I do someone harm so God is punishing me this way?
- Would my beloved husband cheat on me because of this?
- Will I never have kids?

On the first day after returning home from Dr. Ulusoy, these were replaced by,
- This is how I want to raise my child,
- I am normal too,
- I am a woman now,
- I love my husband and he loves me too,
- I can say "I did it" to everyone in the family who knows about this,
- And my legs will no longer tremble. ☺

Or course, I heard the same strong words from my husband too, and believe me, this is the best feeling ever.

Life shouldn't be delayed. The happinesses meant for us need to be experienced. If you can't do it at the time, you need to find the right person and do it.

Those who say it is too far away or who question why they should go to a small town for treatment while living in a big city, please stop creating such excuses and don't delay it. It is much worse to delay because our subconscious is put under more hardship with the treatments, drugs, creams, and sprays that we try to apply by ourselves, or with the stories we hear on the grapevine, or with the unsuccessful treatments we receive.

The brain is the strongest medicine, the brain is the greatest doctor, the brain that can control everything is the most precious consignment from God to us. For three years, I was unable to use my brain for this matter, so I was in need of a helper who could teach me how to use it. And I found that helper. I take this opportunity to thank him once again.

From Trembling Girl with love… / Istanbul

THINGS TO PAY ATTENTION TO DURING FIRST INTERCOURSE

The first night of the marriage is full of question marks for both genders. Women particularly save their first experience for their husbands and the first night of marriage, and until then, they develop protective instincts on that region. At the same time, there is a lack of knowledge regarding the genital area.

The following are advised before the first experience.
1. Together, couples should learn about sex positions and genital areas from books or from the internet.
2. They should read about positive first sexual experience memoirs.

3. They need to get to know about their own naked bodies, as well as that of the other party.
4. They should learn about each other's genital areas within love games and stimulate each other.
5. Rather than abruptly and forcefully penetrating with his penis, the man should start with sensual contact at the inner and outer vagina lips with his penis to create stimulation.
6. When sufficient wetness is obtained, the man should lead his wife toward intercourse without creating any fear or anxiety by helping her take in the tip of the penis first, then half, and then all of it gradually.
7. If there is not enough wetness, they should use lubricant gels.
8. If the penis diameter is larger than the vagina entrance, they should start intercourse by acclimating the vagina first. If necessary, they could try it when the penis is still softer, not in full erection, or they could try different positions to ease penetration.
9. If the woman is describing a stinging or piercing pain at the hymen, they should not force it and see a gynecologist.

The man's knowledgeable and understanding approaches will provide the woman's first sexual experience to happen comfortably.

If there is pain after the first sexual intercourse, it could be due to problems with the hymen or due to dryness. If the woman displays *fear, contraction, panic, pushing her husband away or withdrawal,* she is evaluated as vaginismus, so the couple should not force intercourse and they should apply to a physician working on this subject.

There could be bleeding after the first intercourse. This should not be worrying. It is mostly in the form of leakage. It will diminish and be over until the morning. Very rarely, if the bleeding continues intensively, a gynecologist should be consulted. 40% of the hymens of Turkish women are ring or half-moon shaped. These hymens may not bleed at all and they could allow penetration because they are elastic.

THE RELATIONSHIP BETWEEN THE SEXUAL BRAIN AND SEX LIFE

Below is a quoted passage from Specialist Psychologist Nalan Eyin...

Managing Marriage

According to the data from The European Statistics Office (Eurostat) that shows the divorce rates in European countries, the divorce rate in Turkey has increased 52% between 2007 and 2017.

As per the survey results of Turkish Statistical Institute (TUIK), among the reasons for divorce are gambling, abusing of alcohol, adultery, financial problems, problems with spouse's family and many others. One of the highly rated reason turned out to be *acting irresponsibly and indifferently*.

The rate of women getting divorced due to the man acting irresponsibly and indifferently is 61.5%.

The rate of men getting divorced due to the woman acting irresponsibly and indifferently is 40.2%.

The term of acting irresponsibly and indifferently has a very broad scope. At this section of the book, we will be examining the spouses' responsibilities toward each other in terms of sexuality.

In Turkey, there is the reality of vaginismus cases that are hidden because of embarrassment, as many as there are cases reflected in statistics. Are all the sexual problems between spouses solved after the vaginismus treatment is completed? Unfortunately, no. The differences between the sex life in the man's fantasies and the woman's expectations cause traumas in the inner dynamics of the marriage.

A sexual life that does not provide pleasure will create tension, both individually and also in the communication among spouses. Therefore, the concept of *sexual brain* should be learned and it should be utilized for the more effective management of marriage.

Sexuality is a taboo in our country. Moreover, it is such a taboo that even when people get married and declare each other as spouses, all the negativities related to sex are reflected into the marriage.

Many doyen mental health academicians, experts in their fields, refer to that most important piece in the sustaining of marriage, a piece whose absence is felt, even if they use different words for it. This missing piece, which is introduced as spirituality, attention or affection by the conservative fraction, directly or indirectly emphasizes -in more modernized terms- emotional intelligence and the responsibilities that spouses taken on against each other. We prefer to call this missing piece, or this metaphoric *Holy Grail,* "The Sexual Mind," which comprises all the reasons mentioned here and which indicates much more.

What is meant by the sexual mind is not just the lower brain. It does not point solely at the limbic system, the thrills and emotional reactions. It could be understood as a reference to the relationship between the brain's pleasure zone and the higher cortical activities.

It is difficult to activate the sexual brain for individuals, who do not read, produce, who do not seek meaning in life, who do not love or have occupations.

Now come and let's start by returning to the point where our sexual brains are first shaped as individuals.

Where everything begins; our first home, our family.

Our family passes on much more to us than genes. We can talk about socializing, problem solving, developing empathy, impulse control and sexual education as examples.

As biopsychosocial creatures, beyond the genetic heritage we take, we humans also receive the above-mentioned skills through our families and environmental sources. Parents and other adults that play major roles in the upbringing of a child teach us behavioral patterns that vary from very simple to complex. For instance; smiling, feeling ashamed, sharing your stuff, waiting for your turn, being at peace with others, being sociable, expressing your anger constructively or destructively…

The relationship between the hormones and daily life is truly admirable. For instance, talking and social connections, touching, hugging create an increase of the oxytocin hormone in women. And oxytocin provides the feeling of security as much as it provides feelings of relaxation, tranquility and happiness. So, embrace your woman and establish this behavior not just to impress or flirt, but also to guarantee a long lasting relationship. The wives of men, who don't communicate with their spouses and who don't talk for hours after coming home from work, cannot feed from socializing and they view marriage as a failure. Their inner tension increases, and this tension finds its way to the husband, the actual respondent, like a guided missile. How? As frowning, grunting or leaning toward other social support channels… This is a viscous circle. The disappointed woman starts experiencing this bottomed-out sociality in her relationship, this social hunger, also at the hormonal level.

Her dopamine and oxytocin levels start going down rapidly. This brings along the increase in the stress hormone. And finally the woman becomes unable to cope with the tension created inside her. Our fight or flight responses step in under stress. In such case, the woman will display aggressive impulses that will constantly provide basis for quarrels with her husband, or she will reply with diffidence and alienation.

It is as if the woman, who experiences this in her marriage, is facing an exclusion in her relationship. Evolutionarily, exclusion has been accepted as one of the greatest fears. For humans living in the cave era, being excluded from his tribe or clan was synonymous with death. Because a man had almost zero chance of surviving in the wild nature. Even if our environment has changed, these primal fears are probably still alive beneath the surface. So, no matter how developed and evolved the brain of contemporary man has become, it still operates with the codes inherited from our ancestors.

The human brain is constantly changing and renewing. Although the brain's first development is by genetics and hormones, all our later interactions restructure the brain. So, each daily experience causes the brain's structure to change, to create new neural connections. Isn't it inevitable for the child to eat with his hands if forks and knives are not used in the house? Is it unexpected for a child, whose father yells at the mother with displays of anger, to display his own anger to the people around him with aggression? Or conversely, is it a surprise to expect and observe children from a loving household to reflect the same affection to others?

Undoubtedly, the family, culture and region we are born into are very important factors. But becoming an adult somewhat means being your own software engineer. We need to have the goals of being able to rewrite our own codes, of being individuals that are more effective than the day before and that take more satisfaction from life. And as we are not individuals who live seclusion, we need to succeed in reflecting this to our family, too.

How much pleasure of life could a person have if he is happy on his own but unhappy with his spouse?

Just being well educated, being good-looking and well groomed, having a good occupation and high life standards do not guarantee relationships' success in terms of satisfaction.

Sex on its own cannot keep a relationship above water; that is a fact. Then, is a relationship model that keeps sex alive possible? There, this is exactly the area on which we will be playing our cards.

If the couple has a satisfactory sex life, it means that at least one item on the

Things to Save in Case of Fire list is marked, and that this relationship deserves to be reviewed before termination. This is just like one of the natural things, such as the years we spent for this relationship, the children -if any-, or sharing a mutual history.

When people grow cold of sex, when they cannot get as much pleasure as they used to, they usually question their spouse first. In fact, they also come to seek professional help for this. In the women observation work group that has been going on for almost two and a half years, although a substantial number of women describe themselves as being emotional, approaching their relationship and spouse/partner lovingly, romantically and lustfully, it is clearly visible that what is said and what is done are worlds apart.

Some of the things going on at the women's front are the following.

- **Women are strangers to their own bodies**. Unfortunately this unfamiliarity is not a matter that is proven otherwise by perfectly managing to get into a dress you have bought at a shop without trying it on. This difference should be understood as the difference between knowing the measure of your body and knowing it well enough to analyze its palatal taste. You know very well the tastes that appeal to you while eating, and how you approach sweet, salty or sour tastes. I am talking about applying the same thing on the body.

- **Free-riding tendency**. We are talking about women who expect everything to be perfect and at the peak although they don't exert any effort for sex, just as the impossible phenomenon of a food providing the deliciousness of all spicery although no spice, salt or pepper has been added while cooking it. Sociocultural environment has a very important place. Girls and boys are not raised with the same standards. Being willing, displaying love or behaving warmly even if the man is her husband are factors that are engraved into the minds as making the woman a jezebel. It is a bad thing if the demand for sex comes from the woman, and the woman is even conditioned to refuse whenever such demands comes from the man.

- **The taboo of masturbation**. There are women who cannot touch their own body, who think that they will be sick, lose their virginity or even those who think they will *get pregnant* if they masturbate, as well as women who cannot know what they like or what gives them pleasure.

Then, how can you include these tiny additions that are the spices of the food, into your sex life? The thing that will provide this is the activation of the brain in terms of sex, in other words, by using the sexual brain.

What Kind of Relationship is there between Fear and Orgasm?

Despite being a very cliché phrase, if there is something we know to be absolutely true, it is the fact that the brain is still the greatest and most important sexual organ. Our brain controls sex. This means that a woman is aroused firstly in the brain, not by outer appearance as men are. What does this mean? The amygdala -the fear center of the brain- going on vacation! So, if the amygdala that is the center of fear and tension is active, it is very difficult to have an orgasm. An active amygdala blocks the path to orgasm. *So, while working on the sexual brain, we first need to eliminate the feeling of fear.* (To feel secure and safe.)

In order for orgasm to take place, you first need to feel comfortable, peaceful and relaxed. For instance, imagine that you are relaxing with your feet in hot water. You cannot feel tension and fear while experiencing this feeling. There, this is exactly what the woman needs before sex; to feel truly relaxed and relieved, or even a bit warm! The conditions that will provide relaxation may be formed individually; it is not appropriate to talk about standard lists or must-do rules. As a woman, what are the things that will make you feel relaxed, loosened and cozily warm? Now you can create your own list. Start by writing down a few of them as in the section below. You will see that, in time, you will be able to add other options to the list.

Things that make me relax

1 *(When I...)* ....

2 ....

3 ....

4 ....

5 ....

If you are already feeling relaxed and comfortable, you can help your partner relax even if he has tension himself, and you can even increase your capacity of having an orgasm together.

The sexual brain is the locomotive of sex. It guarantees that you will have an orgasm, increase the duration of your orgasm and take pleasure from the intercourse.

Barry R. Komisaruk and other researchers measured the changes in the women's brains, facial expressions, gestures and body positions at the time of orgasm. Some of the observable findings were shortening of breathing, increase of blood pressure, warm feet, straining of the back, making involuntary sounds. And in their facial expressions, it was seen that they were straining their facial muscles and grimacing as if they were feeling pain. So, it has been scientifically proven with FMRI that orgasm is not just a genital reaction, but that it also creates changes in the brain.

What can we do for the Sexual Brain?

1. **Be in peace with your body**
   Nobody is perfect; don't wait to have a perfect body for a perfect sex. You don't have to look like the *fake* women or men that have been retouched even after professional photo shoots. People, who accept their body for what it is, can relax more easily and their mobility is more elastic.

2. **Don't be afraid to masturbate**
   If you do not know your body, you cannot know what you are capable of doing with it, or what pleasures you could take. You will not be able to lead your partner.

3. **Say no to hearsay information**
   There are plenty of scientific publications and sources in the field of sexual health and anatomy. Investigate. Correct information will prevent you from having groundless anxieties or fears.

4. **Have open communication with your partner**
   Every woman is matchless and unique. Feel free to tell your partner about the things that you personally like, take pleasure from or dislike. If it feels difficult to tell at first, guide him with your hand.

5. **Monotony in sex could end your relationship**
   Include small games into your relationship; be open to try new things. One of the most important magic wands that keep a relationship alive is surprises.

6. **Role-play with your partner**
   These roles are completely meant for discovering pleasure. They are not mandatory but, while role-playing, people feel happy like children playing house. Chain sex and happiness together this way.

7. **Build fantasies**
   Imagination is one of the most important factors that separate humans from other living beings. Fantasies stimulate the sexual brain and enhance it. You can write down these fantasies or you can tell your partner about them.

8. **Actualize the fantasies**

9. **Don't limit sex to just one location**
   As long as your circumstances allow you, don't limit sex to one location. Make use of all the spaces in your home.

10. **Touch**
    Don't forget that men are as sensitive and responsive to touching as women are; reward him with a nice massage.

11. **Pay attention to your thoughts**
    Thoughts turn into emotions, and emotions into behavior. It is not your body that prevents orgasm, but your negative thoughts.

12. **You can develop the sexual brain with hypnotherapy**
    Sexual therapy integrated with hypnotherapy could open the path for taking more pleasure from sex, for being healthy and at peace with yourself, and having relations which are productive and in which you have strong family ties with your spouse.

On the Relationship between the Sexual Brain and Pleasure

Orgasm starts and ends at the brain; the body is merely a tool. The brain is most important among the seven paths that create orgasm.

While the conscious is a limited awareness that can store our current thoughts, i.e. approximately seven units of the information that changes every ten to fifteen seconds, the subconscious is a rich zone.

The past, the now and the future are integrated in the subconscious. The subconscious uses a sui generis encryption and it resembles a concert hall in which millions of information, pictures, memories and fantasies operate simultaneously and in interaction with each other like an orchestra. As the sexual brain evolves, you will start to feel that you are one and whole with everything, you will start taking pleasure from life and as you do, you will also give pleasure to others. Synergy is formed in your relationship.

Developing the sexual brain is not beneficial only for those with sexual dysfunctions, but also for couples that have a normal sex life but that feel distanced from each other due to the dullness and monotony in their relationship. It is the most effective and sustainable key in providing change for those who have never reached orgasm, as well as for those who want to experience orgasm at a heightened level and to prolong the duration of their orgasms.

The younger your brain, the younger you will feel yourself. And your relationship will be young, dynamic, non-monotonous, satisfactory, permanent and loving to the extent that your sexual brain is developed.
Specialist Psychologist Nalan Eyin, September 4, 2020

25 GOLDEN RULES OF NEO-TANTRA ON SEXUALITY

1. Know your own body.
2. Know your partner's body.
3. Know how to give yourself pleasure, whet your pleasures.
4. Know how to give your partner pleasure, whet his/her pleasures.
5. Learn how to discover novelties and differences in sex.
6. Renew yourself in sex.
7. Do not cheat.
8. Live monogamously.
9. Try to give your partner the most possible pleasure.
10. Do not lie to people or to your partner for pleasure.
11. Do not engage in sexual perversions.
12. Follow the nature and the water in sex.
13. Do not harm people for more pleasure.
14. Do not harm your partner for more pleasure.
15. Live sexuality with love and affection.
16. Refrain from loveless, random relationships and sex.
17. Compose a symphony while making love.
18. Dance while making love.
19. Turn lovemaking into a ceremony, a trance.
20. Love nature and the universe, and find them in your partner.
21. Not "Me first" but "You first."
22. Prolong sex.
23. Discover different dimensions of sex.
24. Go beyond sex.
25. Discover and experience sex with a holistic conception of the world.

BREATHING CONTROL

We inhale and exhale from the day we are born. But are we aware of how we are breathing? Shortly, intermittently, sighingly, without letting it all out and by thinking that we are actually breathing... In my twenty-five years of hypnotherapy work since 1990, incorrect breathing is the greatest problem I have observed in my patients. My trainees know that, in The Dr. Ulusoy Hypnosis Induction Technique (Dr. Ulusoy HIT) that I have developed on the basis of this observation, I, as the hypnotherapist, try to arrange the control of breathing with the descent and ascent of my hand at the time of entering hypnosis.

Breathing is key in vaginismus, childbirth, removing obsessive thoughts and behavior in OCD, controlling or stopping the attack in panic attack cases, migraine, Meniere seizures, controlling anger temper tantrums while passing to the evil self in the emotional openings of borderline or impulse control disorders, providing erection and sustaining it, preventing premature ejaculation, concentration, preventing of excitements or the shyness of social phobia, the course of stuttering, self-control, curing of depression, manic-depressive attacks and many other mental illnesses...

The breathing exercises that we give to our patient should be as follows.

1. Inhale slowly and as much as you can, let your lungs fill with air. Imagine them expanding from the bottom to the top, to the edges of each side and inhale without forcing yourself. Hold your breath at the fullest and as much as you are able to without forcing yourself (Within physiological limits). Then exhale slowly. Continue to exhale until your lungs are completely emptied. Do this three to five times a day. Increase the duration that you hold your breath as days and weeks go by.
2. And three to five times in the same day, instead of inhaling and holding your breath, exhale and wait as much as you can without inhaling. Try to prolong this time each day (Within physiological limits).

One and two are separate exercises and they will be done independently. This application, which starts as mini exercises, will be adopted by our subconscious as our new breathing pattern in the following time period. You can do this breathing exercise while walking, sitting, travelling, etc. like a game. After a certain time, without knowing it, your subconscious will adopt this breathing and it will be able to do it without you noticing it.

Our individuality will become stronger and it will be easier for us to fight with mental and physical illnesses. It will also be a prophylactic approach that will prevent the forming of many mental diseases. More importantly, it will make it easier for our conscious/will to reach the subconscious and communicate. Our conscious will be able to make orders with our subconscious.

As a footnote, I would like to remind you that in one of my previous articles, I had mentioned a connection between lifetimes and breathing patterns. I had pointed out that, when the breathing patterns and lifetime of various animals were compared, it was seen that the ones that breathe slowly lived longer.

VAGINAL ORGASM

A considerable number of Turkish women get diagnosed with vaginismus. Fear and anxieties regarding sexuality are in question in vaginismus ethiology, and this is an obstacle for vaginal and clitoral orgasm. Outside of vaginismus, a majority of women are able to experience clitoral orgasms but they are unable to have single or multiple vaginal orgasms. Other than the above, some women can experience neither vaginal nor clitoral orgasm.

Clitoral orgasm is the orgasm that the woman experiences with masturbation in her childhood or teenage years.

For vaginal orgasm, scientists say that the G-spot exists, that it has to exist. But the G-spot has not been exactly located.

Another point of view adopts the thought that vaginal orgasm is formed with mental fantasies.

Another view says that the clitoris is not an organ of pleasure as it is seen from the outside, but that it stands in a way that it surrounds the vagina inside like a horse saddle, and that the penetration and movement of the penis inside the vagina, the squeezing and relaxation or constraint, gives a feeling of pressure and creates vaginal orgasm.

In a research conducted with Doppler and blood stream measurements at the clitoral region, it has been observed that, during vaginal orgasm, the clitoral blood stream increases and the heartrate and blood pressure also increase incrementally. It was also observed that rhythmic convulsions spread throughout the body and that breathing quickens and deepens during vaginal orgasm.

At the end of vaginal orgasm, the woman experiences happiness and relaxation, as well as showing dissociative symptoms such as out of body sensations or looking at her body from above.

Another point of view suggests that vaginal orgasms could be created by strengthening the pubococcygeal pelvic floor muscles with Kegel Exercises.

According to B. Komisaruk, vaginal orgasm occurs at the same place in the brain that is the center of pain and ache. When the facial expression that a woman experiencing vaginal orgasm is examined, a similarity with a painful facial expression is observed. Orgasm also functions as the natural blocker of pain. It can reduce pain up to 50%.

According to our approach, vaginal orgasm is a learnable and developable process. It seems possible for the woman to know -to be taught- what she will experience in vaginal orgasm, for the physiological blood stream and breathing to be directed with suggestion, and for dissociative ego states to be created also with suggestions.

THE ROBOT THEORY

The Psychophysical Reaction Law, also known as *The Robot Theory*, suggests that, for each proposition, thought or emotion that a person has in his mind, there is a corresponding physiological and chemical reaction in his body.

Whatever the mind believes or whichever reality it accepts, the body obeys it like a robot. Reality is not singular for the mind. The reality of each individual varies according to his experiences in life.

This is a great explanation for those who ask how it is possible for hypnosis to have somatic effects. Neuropsychobiology investigates this situation with all details. But for centuries, shamans and psychologists have been using hypnosis without knowing the mechanism and they still are.

Another citation from Ibn-Sina says, "Imagination exists in humans. Not only can this imagination heal illnesses, it can also create illnesses out of nothing."

And I say, "The mind does what it imagines and believes. The rest are details for the mind!"

GENITO-PELVIC PAIN OR PENETRATION DISORDER (DSM 5 TR) DIAGNOSIS SCALE

Signs and symptoms of genito-pelvic pain/penetration disorder include persistent or recurrent difficulties with one (or more) of the following:
1. Vaginal penetration during intercourse.
2. Marked vulvovaginal or pelvic pain during vaginal intercourse or penetration attempts.

Marked fear or anxiety about vulvovaginal or pelvic pain in anticipation of, during, or as a result of vaginal penetration.

Marked tensing or tightening of the pelvic floor muscles during attempted vaginal penetration.

To be diagnosed with genito-pelvic pain/penetration disorder, a patient's symptoms must be present for at least six months and cause clinically significant distress. Also, the sexual dysfunction should not be better explained by a nonsexual mental disorder or as a consequence of a severe relationship distress (e.g. partner violence) or other significant stressors, nor be attributable to the effects of a substance/medication or another medical condition.

Check for the existence of the following.

- Lifelong: This dysfunction has been there since the person has become sexually active.
- Acquired: This dysfunction has begun after a rather ordinary sexual functionality period.

Indicate the intensity at the time.
- Non-intensive: The symptoms above create minor distress.
- Intermediate: The symptoms above create a medium-level distress.
- Severe: The symptoms above create major distress.

Note: The DSM 5 TR diagnosis scale for vaginismus has been included for therapists. When you check our definitions of vaginismus at the beginning of the book, you can clearly see the cultural differences. This is why there are differences in its causes and treatments, as there are differences in the diagnosis and definitions that are derived from literature and from our experiences.

We had begun our book with a story, let's end with another...

TRUE LOVE STORIES - 2

In our first story, we said that true love was a feeling that comes from the heart. Most of the time, true loves are perhaps condemned to remain platonic. Many people love but the other party cannot love them back because they see love in other elements, or the loving party cannot express themselves with words. Maybe they can even hurt you with their words without meaning to do so.

Showing Mimar Sinan[12] and Mihrimah Sultan[13] as example[14], I asked this in one of my trainings, "Why do you think that all the passionate one-sided or mutual loves in history and mythology have ended in disappointment, separation or without getting together?" The answer was just as appropriate, "Because if they had been together, it wouldn't have been called love..."

It was a very accurate determination. And when we look at poets, writers, sculpturers or painters, we see that there is the existence of a passionate love or separation behind all those beautiful works of art. This love could be the love of God, as well as the love for a sweetheart. And the artists engrave this passion into their pieces of art. This engraving process brings out the beauty of the piece.

---

(12) **TN:** Mimar Sinan was the chief Ottoman architect and civil engineer, also known as *Sinan Agha the Grand Architect.*

(13) **TN:** Mihrimah Sultan was an Ottoman princess. She was the most powerful imperial princess in Ottoman history.

(14) **TN:** Mimar Sinan was hopelessly in love with Mihrimah Sultan. His love for her was desperate, never to be, but he expressed it in his artwork, building two mosques in her name that are considered among the pinnacles of Ottoman architecture.

Apparently, when people are in a passionate love and/or when they are unable to get together, a special state of consciousness is created in their subconscious. This state of consciousness triggers creativity and inspiration.

Had Mevlana not expressed his love for Shams and for God in his Masnavi?

Sezai Karakoç defines this love in his wonderful verse,
"Shams was a question
An answer Mevlana was
Together they resembled
A conversation one had with himself"
And see the wonderful metaphor Mevlana has used for love in his Fîhi Ma-Fîh.

"Majnun wanted to write a letter to Layla[15]; he took a pen and said this verse:
Your vision is before my eyes, your name is in my mouth, your memory is in my heart, where should I write?
Since your vision has settled in the eye, your name does not leave my mouth, your memory is in my house of life,
Then, to whom should I write the letter? You are already all around.
He said and broke the pen, tore the paper."

True loves and affections are mostly invisible. How could you see your love for God? But God is reflected on humans, creatures and the universe so that you can see him. Through His creations, we can see His activity of creating, His love, grace, art and His perfect order...

This is why love cannot be expressed with words. It reflects on behaviors, thoughts, actions and creations. Maybe he cannot say, "I love you," but he can make you feel that love. Just as God has all those beautiful names, He also has names that are agonizing. And man is a whole of all these names. He is us and we are He...

We have good sides and bad sides too. We try to mature over the years in fits and starts; sometimes hurting others unintentionally, sometimes making them happy. The important thing is to increase our good deeds in the scale

---

(15) **TN:** In the famous poem/story, Qays and Layla fall in love with each other when they are young, but when they grow up Layla's father doesn't allow them to be together. Qays becomes obsessed with her, and his tribe and the community give him the epithet of Majnun (Possessed by Jinn).

of balance, and to make the perfections in our essence visible and noticeable without being outcast because of our bad doings.

The key point of living long-lasting loves and relationships with affection, peace and happiness:

In relationships, we may display sudden reactiveness that originate from the shadows in our subconsciouses and that could cause arguments, resentments, anger, rage or estrangements. Both in friendships and marriages, the key for the friendship, love and affection to be sustained for many years is to be aware of our reactions that do not reflect our essence, that come from our shadows. *Our reactions that originate from our shadows never reflect our true self...* Whatever happens in life, as loyal individuals, it is important for us to remember the good sides of the person across from us, to act as mirrors to support each other's mental development, and to keep true lovers and friends around us. Because true lovers and friends are rare. They are with you through your good and bad days; you should not lose them...

"There are people
They come and pass through our lives...
Some go with earthquakes, some with storms...
I support the ones that stay...
I like the loyalty and patience of the ones that stay..."

Shams Tabrizi

And a final word...

The book "Hypnosis for Vaginismus Treatment & the Importance of Psoas Muscles" is a product of my endeavor -with years of passionate love- on solving the vaginismus problem with hypnotherapy. You have read brief and practical ways for vaginismus treatment...

March 29, 2015 – Dr. Ulusoy, Kuşadası, 9:30 p.m.

"Whatever you do, do it with love, and give people happiness by doing the best in everything in life."

CHAPTER 6

REFERENCES AND PHOTOGRAPHS

REFERENCES

- The Power of Myth, J. Campbell, Mediacat Publications
- Evaluation, Diagnosis and Treatments in Two Frequent Sexual Dysfunctions: Vaginismus and Premature Ejaculation, Asst. Prof. Psych. Ceylan Tuğrul
- Sexual Behavior Disorders, Prof. Psych. Adnan Ziyalar
- Hypnotherapy in Sexual Problems, Psych. Tahir Özakkaş
- Holotropic Breathwork, S. Grof, Ray Publications
- Spiritual Emergency, S. Grof, Kaknüs Publications
- The Book of Pain, Dr. Serdar Erdine, Hayy Publications
- Sex Therapy, Dr. Cebrail Kısa
- Completely Overcome Vaginismus, Mark – Lisa Carter
- Sexual Reflexology, Mantak Chia, Dharma Publications
- www.tantraakademi.com, Dr. Ümit Sayın
- Breathing Therapy, Mustafa Kartal, Ray Publications
- HypnoBirthing from The Wizard Within, Dr. Al Krazner, Gün Publishing
- DSM V TR, Diagnosis Criteria, Translator: Prof. Ertuğrul Köroğlu, Physicians Publications Union
- The Sufi and the therapist, Facebook page, Sezai Karakoç

PHOTOGRAPHS

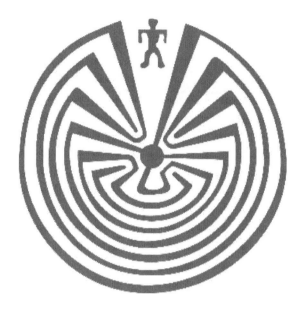

The above logo is a registered logo that symbolizes The Dr. Ulusoy Therapy Approach and Hypnosis Applications.

The point at the middle connotes the inner source. The rings around it are the different states of consciousness. The Dr. Ulusoy Therapy Approach is problem-based and it indicates the human figure reaching its inner sources directly and solving the problem with his inner *Intelligent Mind – Subconscious*. "No problem can be solved from the same level of consciousness that created it," says Einstein, and he is right. In order to solve the problem, we need to go deeper than the consciousness level that has created it and to the altered states of consciousness (Trance). By utilizing hypnosis in our therapies, we reach the inner course and we work on emotions by interacting with the subconscious via symbols, archetypes and ideomotor. We create new neuronal paths directed toward affections and new learnings. This new formation starts to change thoughts, behaviors and somatic (Bodily) structures like *the bushing out and growing of the seeds that have been planted in thoughts.*

This logo also expresses an archetypic symbol that belonged to the Indians.

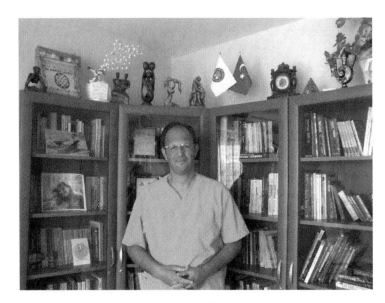

Dr. Murat Ulusoy

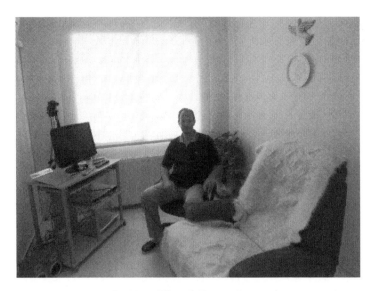

Dr. Murat Ulusoy's Therapy Room

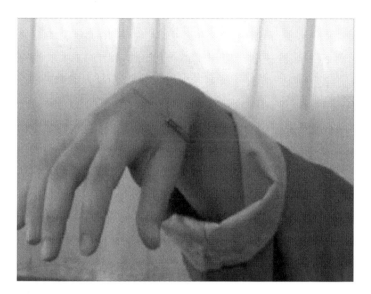

Creating a pain-free area at the back of the hand with suggestions under hypnosis and sticking a needle. Photo taken from Hypnosis Inductions Training CD, 2001

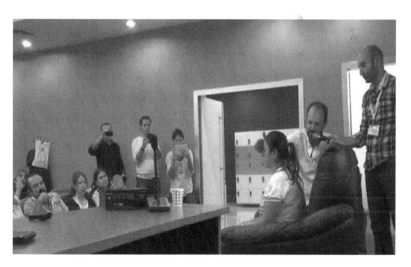

Dr. Ulusoy Hypnosis Induction Technique, from Üsküdar University Medical Hypnosis Training, 2014

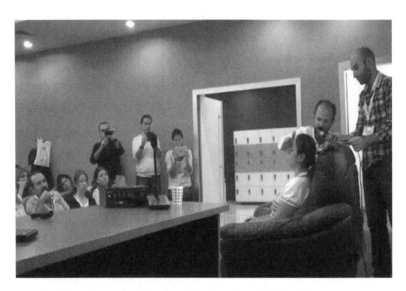

Dr. Ulusoy Hypnosis Induction Technique, from Üsküdar University
Medical Hypnosis Training, 2014

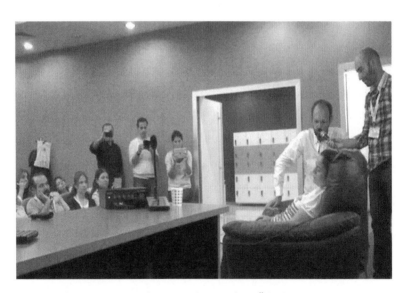

Dr. Ulusoy Hypnosis Induction Technique, from Üsküdar University
Medical Hypnosis Training, 2014

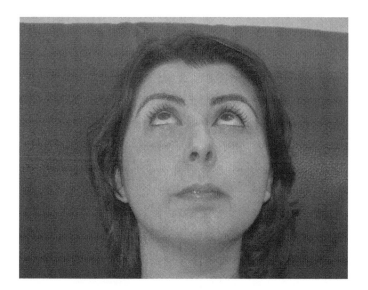

Aptitude test for looking up. Enacting with Aksu E.B. to demonstrate induction. Photo by Funda Ulusoy, 2015

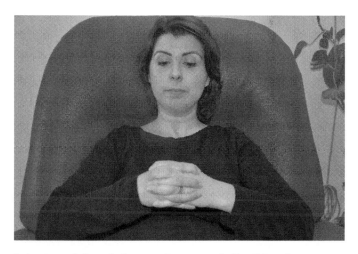

Induction with finger locking test. Enacting with Aksu E.B. to demonstrate induction. Photo by Funda Ulusoy, 2015

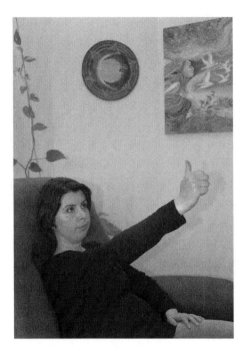

Eye Fixation Induction Technique. Enacting with Aksu E.B. to demonstrate induction. Photo by Funda Ulusoy, 2015

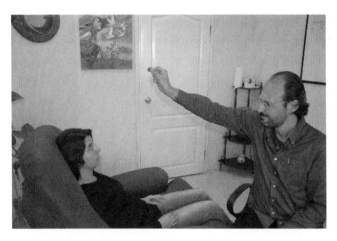

Braid's Inductions Application. Enacting with Aksu E.B. to demonstrate induction. Photo by Funda Ulusoy, 2015

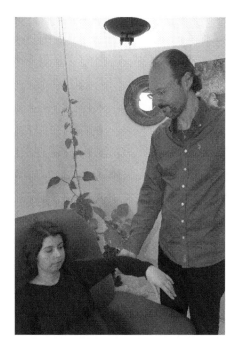

Induction with arm dropping test. Enacting with Aksu E.B. to demonstrate induction. Photo by Funda Ulusoy, 2015

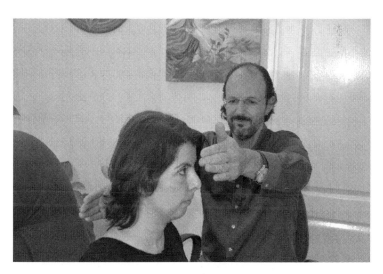

Dr. Ulusoy Hypnosis Induction Technique. Enacting with Aksu E.B. Photo by Funda Ulusoy, 2015

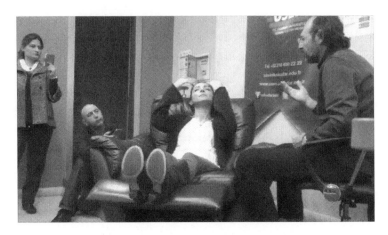

Ideomotor Effect and Influencing the Subconscious. Photo from hypnosis training at Üsküdar University, 2015

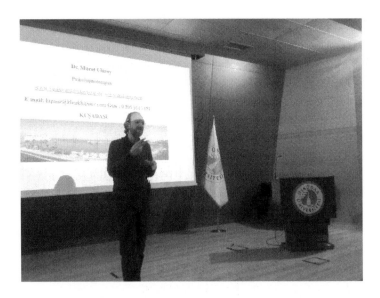

Istanbul Medical Hypnosis Congress, Üsküdar University, 2014

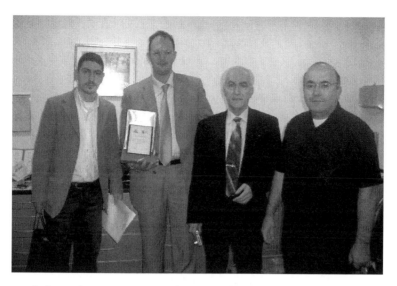

Left to right: Hüsnü Müezzinoğlu, Murat Ulusoy, Ali Eşref Müezzinoğlu, Tahir Özakkaş at Yeditepe University, 2004

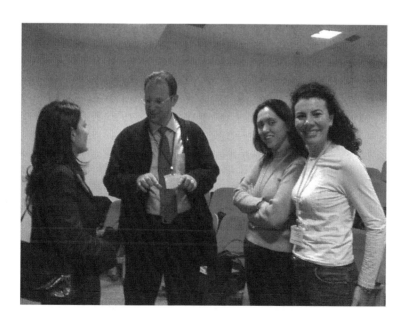

Yeditepe University, Break during training, 2003

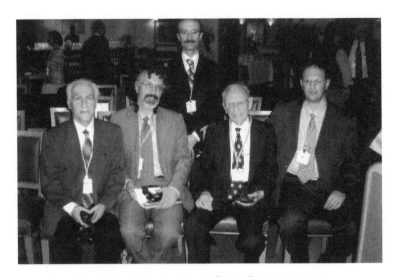

Left to right: Ali Eşref Müezzinoğlu, Ali Özden Öztürk, Haluk Alan,
John G. Watkins, Murat Ulusoy

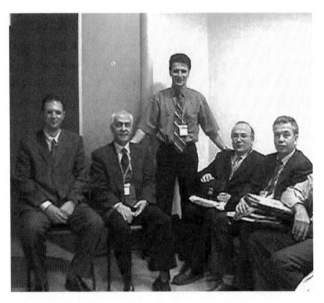

Left to right: Murat Ulusoy, Ali Eşref Müezzinoğlu, Tuncay Özer,
Tahir Özakkaş, Kemal Nuri Özerkan during the Medical Hypnosis
Congress at Yeditepe University

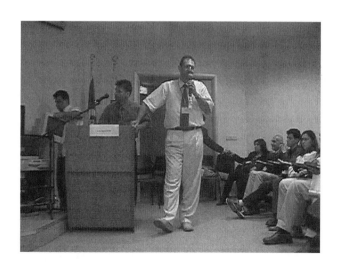

12th European Hypnosis Congress (ESH), 2011

Medical Hypnosis Training at Yeditepe University, 2002

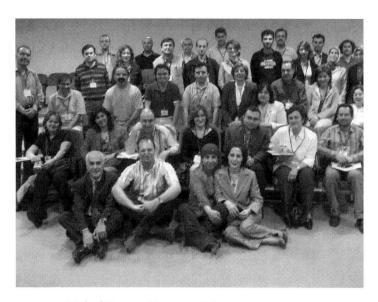

Medical Hypnosis Training at Yeditepe University, 2003

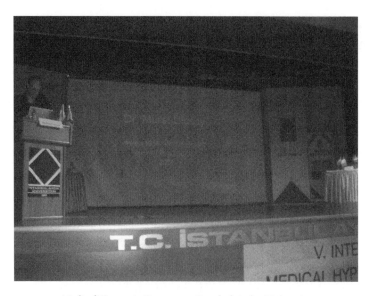

Medical Hypnosis Congress at Istanbul Aydın University

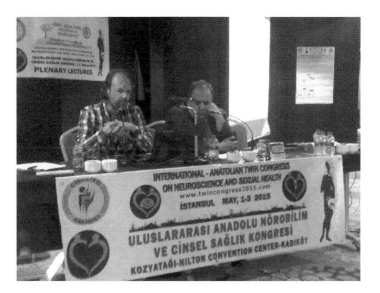

Dr. Murat Ulusoy and Prof. Dr. Ümit Sayın at the 1st Anatolian Neuroscience and Sexual Health Congress, 2015

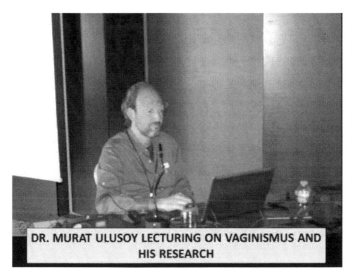

Dr. Murat Ulusoy at the 1st Anatolian Neuroscience and Sexual Health Congress, 2015

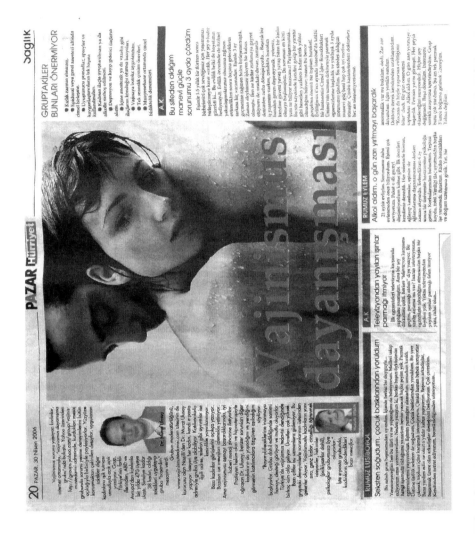

Our free support on Vaginismus Treatment Yahoo! Group was reported as news by Mesude Erşan in the Hürriyet Newspaper on April 30, 2006

RUMUZ AYCA

6'ncı ayımıza gerçekten karı-koca gireceğiz

D, ben şu anda tek parmak 2,5-3 boğum aşamasındayım. Belki bu akşam 2 parmağı deneyeceğim. Başarınlar çok olunca azim geldi. Ben de dün itibariyle 5 aylık evliyim. İnşallah 6'ncı ayımıza gerçekten karı-koca olarak girmiş oluruz. Desteklerinizi bekliyorum. En kısa zamanda kocaman harflerle "başardım" yazmak dileğiyle...

İSİMSİZ

Kendini sıkma yapabileceğine inan

E, bak, "Vajinama bakmak bile çok zor geliyor" diyordun. Artık bakabiliyorsun. Eğer parmak egzersizlerine başlayamıyorsan sadece elinle vajinanı tanımaya çalış. Kendini hazır hissettiğinde başlarsın egzersizlere. Acele yok. Panik ve ben yapamayacağım da yok. Eğer bu siteyi bulduysan ve gruba eklendiysen başarı yarıya yavaş yavaş gelecek inan buna. Kendini sıkma, sadece yapabileceğine inan. Kolay gelsin arkadaşım.

İSİMSİZ

Acele edersen başa dönersin

A, seni anlıyorum. Diğer arkadaşlar gibi, bir an önce "başardım" diye yazmak istiyorsun. Başaracaksın ama tek parmağın hepsi girmeden ve en az bir hafta denemeden 2 parmağa geçme, derin arkadaşım. Tamamen rahat olduğunda, 2 parmağa geçtiğinde hem daha rahat edersin hem de sağlam adımlarla ilerlemiş olursun. Acele edersen bir şeyler eksik kalırsa tekrar başa dönebilirsin.

A.K.

Bir adım atarsan gerisi gelecek

E, bu aşamaları bu sitedeki tüm kadınlar gibi hepimiz yaşadık. Umutsuz, yenik, yıkılmış günlerin olması çok normal. Ama inan bir kez daha adım atarsan gerisi de gelecek. Bu egzersizde en önemli adım önce tek parmak, tek boğum ve sonra da iki parmak bir boğum aşaması. Bu iki adımı atlatabilirsen şöyle bir geriye doğru baktığında öyle küçülür ki, sen de şaşırırsın.

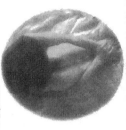

RUMUZ ASYA

Ölmeden sorunumu halletmek istiyorum

Tek parmak 2.5 boğumdayım. 15 dakikadan fazla çalışamıyorum. Sitenin sanırım en yaşlı ve en kronik vakasıyım. Uzun süreli evliliğimi cinsellik yaşamadan bitirdim. Evliliğimin ilk gecesi hamile kalıp çocuk sahibi olmuş ve hiç birleşmeyi yaşamamış biriyim. Şu an bir partnerim var ve sık görüşemiyorum. Ben de kendi kendime, ölmeden bu sorunumu halletmeyi karar verdim.

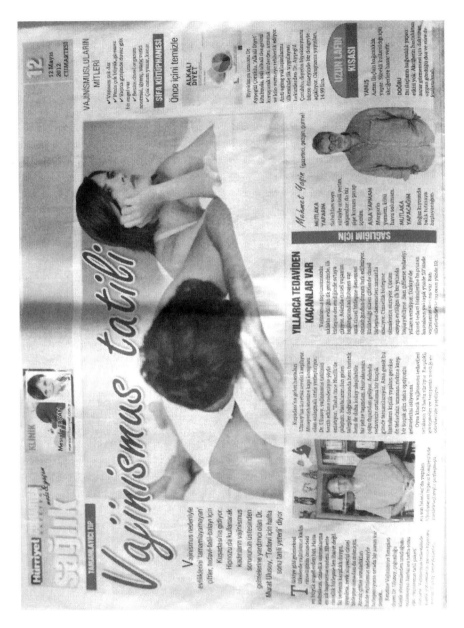

The Dr. Ulusoy Method in vaginismus treatment. Our patients, who reach results in one and a half days, come to Kuşadası for both treatment and honeymoon. One weekend is enough for treatment. Mesude Erşan's news on Hürriyet Newspaper

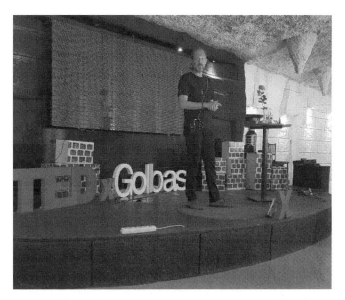

Tedxgolbasi, Vaginismus treatment and social responsibility, 2018

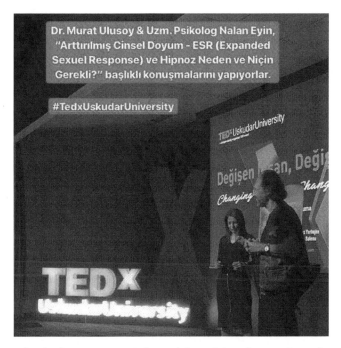

Tedxuskudaruniversity, Enhanced Sexual Satisfaction, Specialist Psychologist Nalan Eyin and Dr. Murat Ulusoy, 2019

DAY-2
ULUSOY

2. INTERNATIONAL ANATOLIAN CONGRESS
ON NEUROSCIENCE AND SEXUAL HEALTH
İSTANBUL   NOVEMBER 16-17   2019
KOZYATAĞI-HILTON TWIN TOWERS

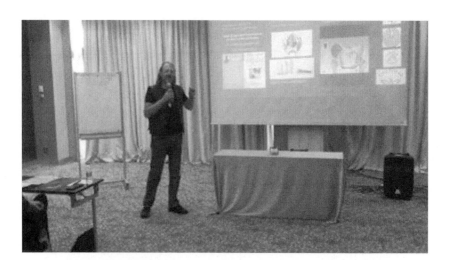

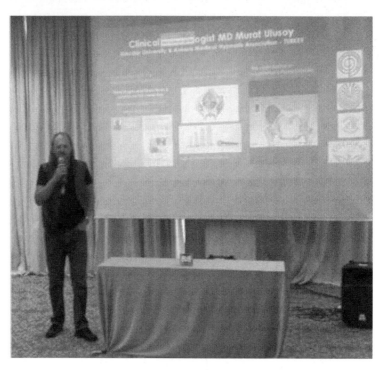

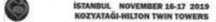

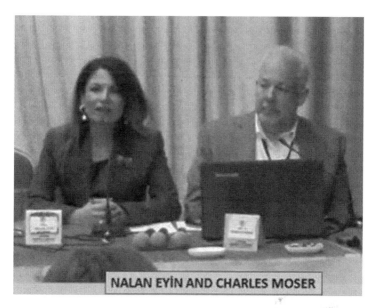

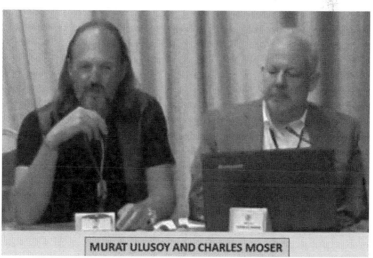

Prof. Charles Moser and Dr. Murat Ulusoy at the International Anatolian
Neuroscience and Sexual Health Congress, 2019

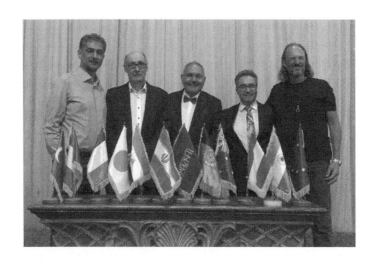

Dr. Mehdi Fathi, Ish President Bernhard, Dt. Murat Uslu, Dr. Shahidi,
Dr. Murat Ulusoy at Asia Hypnosis Congress in Iran, 2019

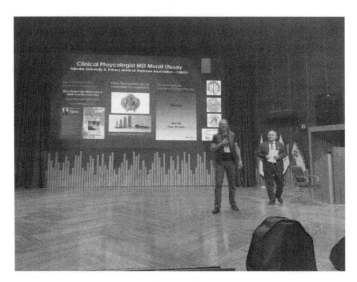

Asia Hypnosis Congress in Iran, 2019

Printed in Great Britain
by Amazon

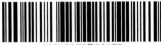